90 Days to Beautiful Hair: 50 Dermatologist-Approved Tips to Un"lock" The Hair of Your Dreams

90 Days to Beautiful Hair: 50 Dermatologist-Approved Tips to Un"lock" The Hair of Your Dreams

Crystal Aguh, MD

ISBN-13: 978-0-578-50226-7

DEDICATION

This book is dedicated to my loving husband, Chike, and our son, Kelechi. Thank you both for inspiring me to share my thoughts with the world.

Contents

Introduction

Why I Wrote This Book

I f you are reading this book, it is likely that you have found yourself disappointed with the state of your hair. Maybe you underwent three rounds of chemotherapy and no longer recognized the hair you were born with and have become frustrated. Or perhaps you have started to notice that your trusted ponytail holder now wraps around your ponytail a few more times than it did in the past. Regardless of what brought you here, thank you for coming; and I hope that you find precisely what you are looking for in this book: a road map to healthier, longer, stronger hair.

People always ask me how I came up with the idea of writing this book. Well, it's because I have spent most of my life struggling with my own hair care. Growing up, my mom, who worked long hours, found it much easier to style me and my sister's hair in ways that would require the least amount of upkeep and effort. That meant frequent relaxers (starting at age 5) and the use of extensions. I had extensions almost consistently until I turned 28. As a dermatologist-in-training, I saw many women coming in with complaints of hair loss. And, just like recommendations on the best sunscreen, I quickly learned that it would be helpful to figure out a handful of products to recommend for hair care.

The hard part was, these recommendations were nowhere to be found. They were not in dermatology textbooks, and they were certainly not a part of dermatology training. I began experimenting with my own hair care, delving into YouTube tutorials and trying multiple products, reading and dissecting scientific studies on best practices. Through all this, I eventually got to the point where I felt comfortable teaching other dermatologists about hair care. Fast forward a couple of years and I was convinced by a colleague to write a book about hair care, the first of its kind written by and for dermatologists. I have spent the years since, delivering talks around the country about the best hair care practices to help our hair thrive.

No matter how many times I give my talk, one line always generates the disbelief:

The principles for healthy hair care are the same, regardless of hair type.

This is a mind-blowing concept for most people. The fact of the matter is, most of the labels that we put on our hair are designed by companies for marketing purposes only and have no bearing on what actually works best for your hair. The true determinant of what will work best for you is based on the ingredients that make up your hair product. So, if you are a brunette and buy a shampoo meant for blondes, nothing bad will happen. I promise. And if you are a black woman with tightly curled hair and use a shampoo outside of the "ethnic hair" aisle, the same concept applies, you will be just fine.

Of course, there are different hair colors and curl patterns, but the chemical structure of all hair is the same, and for the most part, hair thrives under the same conditions. For some hair types, namely curly hair, near-ideal hair practices are needed for the hair to achieve maximum lengths and fullness.

While hair grows an average of a ½ inch per month, there are some differences in growth rates between ethnic groups (Asian hair grows slightly faster than that, and African hair slightly slower) and the curl patterns also varies widely among racial and ethnic groups.

One of the main reasons that curly hair requires more care is because it is less likely to be coated with sebum. Sebum is a natural moisturizer produced by the scalp and works to protect the hair strand from damage. A single brush stroke can coat the entire hair strand in women with straight or wavy hair leading to hair that stays stronger, for a longer period of time. For people with curly hair, the sebum gets stuck near the scalp, unable to make it down all of the twists and turns of tightly curled hair. Couple this with the fact that the growth rate of the hair in many women of African descent is slightly slower, and the result is that it is harder for many curly haired black women to grow their hair past shoulder length.

The good news is that with the right instruction and a healthy hair regimen, anyone can unlock their hair's maximum potential and reach lengths they may not have ever deemed possible.

Here is what this book will not do:

- It will not give you a super-secret tip to making your hair grow faster, even if you can get it to grow longer. How fast your hair grows is determined by your DNA and cannot be altered. Certainly, if I discover how to change your pre-determined genetic growth rate, I will write a book for all of my loyal readers and retire somewhere on an island far, far away.
- It will not change the natural characteristics of your hair. So, while this healthy hair care regimen may lead to fuller hair over time, this is due to less breakage and not because your naturally fine hair suddenly became thick. Depending on who you are, this change may still be drastic, especially if you have hair that is currently very damaged.

So, what will this book do?

- Give you healthy alternatives for your favorite styling practices
- Provide you with a list of ingredients to look for in your hair products to make shopping easier
- Teach you how to improve the strength of your hair and prevent further damage
- Help you devise a unique hair regimen specifically tailored to what your hair needs

Some women will have to pay closer attention to the tips in this book than others. That is because the more tender loving care (TLC) your hair requires, the smaller the margin for error. The amount of TLC your hair needs is based on your hair type and the amount of damaging treatments to which it has been subjected. Not sure where you fall on the TLC curve? Well here's a helpful diagram:

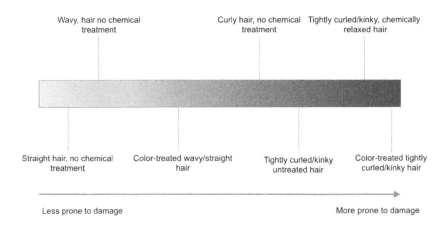

This diagram can help you understand just how many tips you will need to incorporate into your regimen. Of course, it does not take into account all of the different types of hair that are out there but should give a general sense of how prone to damage your hair can be. While heat styling is not noted on this diagram, regular heat styling can be as damaging as chemically processing the hair, and you should approach it as such.

As you read this book, keep in mind where your hair falls on the TLC curve. If you are further to the right, be prepared to make at least a handful of adjustments before seeing any improvement, but also realize that the potential upside is greatest at this side of the curve.

Lastly, while incorporating these tips should lead to some immediate improvements, if you are serious about restoring your optimum health, then you should plan on incorporating these tips for the foreseeable future. If you follow these tips just once, you will notice no long-term benefit. Hair is not living tissue, so once it is damaged, it cannot repair itself. At a growth rate of ½ inch per month, it means that if you want to grow 12 inches of healthy hair, you will need, on average, two years of consistency to reach your goal. In the end, however, it will all be completely worth it.

Be patient. Be open-minded. Be prepared to unlock the hair of your dreams.

One

Ignore the Labels on Hair Products

To fully absorb the tips that you will read in this book, you will have to be prepared to let go of some of your assumptions about hair care. I have learned that one of the hardest things to do, is to get people to think outside the box when it comes to hair. This is especially important when it comes to product marketing labels.

I'll never forget the time I stayed with a close friend of mine, who is a brunette, while I was writing this book. She asked me to go over her hair care regimen and give her tips on hair care since she was experiencing recurrent damage from flat ironing her hair every day. I noticed in her bathroom that she had two brands of shampoo and conditioner, one containing the ingredients found in this book, and the other containing more damaging ingredients I encourage avoiding. Well turns out, the "good" shampoo belonged to her roommate, a blonde, and had been marketed to people with dyed hair. She was shocked when I told her she did not need dyed hair to try it, and she noticed immediate results after one use.

Similarly, many of my black patients have recommended products that they have found outside of the "ethnic hair" aisle and have been amazed at how well they worked for them.

It is time to think outside of the box.

Hair companies realize that marketing their products to specific demographics can make patients feel "special" when in reality it's just a ploy.

When searching for hair products, you should feel comfortable ignoring these marketing ploys and pay attention to the ingredients that are safe for your hair. Generally speaking, products marketed toward "ethnic hair," and those marketed as "color safe" tend to have gentle, less damaging ingredients than those marketed toward other hair types, so this is not a bad place to start when looking for products. This is because hair that is curly and hair that has been colored are more prone to damage and require more TLC. However, there are also plenty of products marketed toward these groups that have damaging ingredients and are misleading, so you will still need to be on alert.

Those with curly and/or colored hair should also feel comfortable branching out and trying products that are not marketed to them. Unfortunately, very few people are armed with the knowledge necessary to choose products that make sense for them, and that is a crucial goal of this book. By the time you are finished reading, you should feel comfortable walking down any beauty aisle and choosing the products that make the most sense for you.

Two

Don't Go Broke Buying Expensive Products

The beauty aisle in any pharmacy or grocery store is a beautiful array of multicolored hair products meant to appeal to the aesthetic inclinations of women everywhere. I have personally been known to reach and grab the products with the most beautiful packaging, especially when I knew less about what to look for on the ingredients label. Back then, I also spent a lot of money just out of a pure desire to try as many products as possible, even when I had products at home that worked just fine. It was almost like an addiction. I had become a certified "product junkie."

After reading this book, I want to urge you to avoid the desire to purchase tons of products. If this is the first time that you are going to try to "go healthy" regarding your hair care, keep a few things in mind before you go to the hair store:

1. Go to the store with a plan. Check out non-biased sources for recommendations on products for your hair type and research the ingredients online. Every woman, especially if your hair is dry or damaged, should have a reliable product from each of the following categories:
    *   Shampoo
    *   Rinse out conditioner
    *   Leave-in conditioner/daily moisturizer
    *   Deep Conditioner

Start with these "core four" products and then go on from there. If your hair is really damaged and you need a protein conditioner, add that too. Don't get hypnotized with things like 'smoothing oil,' 'hair nutrient complex' and other fancy-sounding products. Just stick with the basics.

2. Use the ingredients listed in this book to help guide your product selection. If you find the perfect shampoo for you and its $2, then great, you're all set!

3. Resist the temptation to buy products just because they are expensive; they still may be damaging to your hair. Obviously, there are some expensive products that are quite amazing, but do your research first and don't be guided by price alone.

4. Be patient! It may take months, even a couple of years, before you find the right set of products for your hair, but if you're not satisfied, keep looking. The ideal shampoo should leave your hair feeling clean, but not dry. The ideal deep conditioner should make your hair feel nice and soft and allow it to retain that level of moisture for at least a few days.

Three

Determine Your Ideal Shampooing Frequency

Shampooing and conditioning is the cornerstone of any healthy hair regimen. The first step in building your hair care routine is determining your ideal washing frequency. This is an important question because hair-washing is not a one size fits all type of routine. Sebum, the moisturizer produced from our scalp, really likes to attract dirt. It has a much easier time coating straight strands than wavy or curly strands. As a result, people with straight hair may notice their hair feeling limp and oily within 24 hours of their last shampooing. Women with really curly hair often have an issue with their hair feeling too dry, mainly because sebum has a harder time moving down the length of curly hair. For this reason, curly hair does not feel dirty as quickly as straight hair and also takes longer to feel limp. As such, it does not require frequent washing.

Shampooing is a "necessary evil." It cleans the hair, but by stripping away the hair's sebum, it also leaves it in a vulnerable state. Before you embark on your plan to optimize your hair regimen, you will need to optimize your shampooing frequency. If you have long, straight hair but are suffering from breakage, you can try washing your hair every other day instead of every day or alternating between a regular shampoo + conditioner and washing with conditioner alone (see Chapter 9).

Those with wavy hair may be able to get away with washing their hair 2–3 times per week, while those with curly hair may shampoo as little as once every 1–2 weeks. Sometimes this changes as the seasons change and you may find that shampooing your hair more often is a must in the summertime, while you can get away with longer shampooing intervals during the winter months. Try to always pay attention to the signals your hair is giving you and remain flexible.

I generally recommend that those with fine, straight hair shampoo their hair once daily predominately with a sulfate-free cleanser (see Chapter 4), and those with tightly curled hair shampoo a *minimum* of once every two weeks. I do not recommend going longer than that between shampoos because deep conditioners and protein treatments tend to work better on freshly washed hair.

Are you considering adding a dry shampoo to your regimen? Dry shampoos work well to sop up sebum and often contain ingredients like cornstarch or rice starch. Incorporating dry shampoos can be useful for occasional use, as they avoid the damage that can occur from re-wetting the hair, but will not remove heavier oils left on by styling products. However, over time, the ingredients from dry shampoo build up and may require removal with a harsher shampoo to clean the hair so I would not recommend them for curly hair.

Four

Start Using a Sulfate-Free Shampoo and Learn How to Spot One

I believe that a healthy hair care regimen begins with a proper cleansing regimen, especially for women with damaged hair. As I mentioned in the previous chapters, sebum is a natural hair protectant produced by the scalp. Sebum does a great job at moisturizing the hair and protecting it from everyday wear and tear. While it's essential to make sure your hair is clean, it's best not to do it at the expense of removing all of the natural sebum from the hair strand. To help understand where your shampoo ingredients come into play, it's important to know how shampoos work.

The earliest shampoos used on the hair were basic soaps that people used on their skin. These were not meant to have any properties to beautify the hair and certainly did not make the hair appear any glossier. Their most basic function was, and still is, to remove dirt from the hair. We no longer use basic soaps to wash our hair and instead, we use more complex shampoos, many of which contain multiple types of cleansing ingredients as well as conditioning agents and glossers to please the consumer.

All shampoos are composed of at least one basic ingredient called a surfactant. A surfactant is designed to be attracted to both dirt and water, allowing dirt to be washed out easily while bathing. There are many different types of surfactants marketed today, but they generally fall into one of four classes: anionic, cationic, non-ionic, and amphoteric. Don't worry, I know most of you have nightmares from your chemistry class, so I will keep this brief and limit it only to what you need to know to keep your hair beautiful.

ANIONIC SURFACTANTS

The most common surfactant used is an anionic surfactant. In fact, almost all ingredients listed on your shampoo that contain the word "-sulfate" are anionic surfactants. This type of surfactant is superb at removing dirt from the hair making it ideal for cleansing. Unfortunately, anything great at removing dirt is often great at removing protective sebum as well. For those with straight hair, this is not much of an issue because sebum is produced daily and can recoat the hair quickly, but for curly or damaged hair thirsting for moisture, it can lead to less than desirable results.

Anionic surfactants get their name from the fact that they are negatively charged. Our hair hates a negative charge, and when shampoo is applied to the hair, the negative charge is left behind. So if you forget to use a conditioner, you will notice hair that is dry, brittle and frizzy. To restore the hair's neutral charge, a conditioner, which is positively charged, is required. This is the reason why the two must be used together, and shampoo cannot be used alone. I generally recommend that my patients with damaged hair, of any type, try and minimize their use of shampoos that have harsh anionic surfactants but I will explain more below.

SULFATE-FREE SHAMPOOS

So how can you determine if your shampoo is sulfate-free? You can start by looking at the bottle- most sulfate free shampoos will put a label on the front of the bottle. However, just because the bottle says sulfate free does not mean it does not contain harsh ingredients, and this is where it gets tricky.

The most commonly used anionic surfactant, sodium lauryl sulfate (SLS), is considering the prototypical member of the 'sulfate' class and is also believed to have the best cleansing ability. Likewise, it is also considered to be the harshest of all shampoo surfactants. This can be problematic, not only for women with curly hair but also for those with hair that has been heat-damaged, has been colored or chemically styled.

Often, when companies label their shampoos as "sulfate-free," they are referring to the absence of SLS. However, many other anionic surfactants can be nearly as damaging as SLS, including sodium laureth sulfate (SLES) or ammonium laureth sulfate (ALS). Sometimes shampoos will label themselves as sulfate-free if they are missing just SLS and sometimes they will call themselves sulfate free if they are just missing any one of these three, there really is no standard.

I have a much higher standard when considering if a shampoo is sulfate free and that is whether or not it contains an anionic surfactant. Again, most of my patients are suffering from severe hair damage, and even the gentler anionic surfactants can be too harsh for their hair.

If you are committed to avoiding sulfate-containing shampoos, specifically those free of anionic surfactants, please refer to the table below for a list of ingredients to look for. Take this with you when you go to the beauty supply store or pharmacy and shop for your favorite shampoos:

Anionic Surfactants
The products are the best at removing product buildup but can be drying. Use sparingly (listed from most harsh to least harsh)
Sodium Lauryl Sulfate Sodium Laureth Sulfate Sodium Lauroyl Sarcosinate Ammonium Lauryl Sulfate Sodium Myreth Sulfate Sodium C14-16 Olefin Sulfonate Disodium laureth sulfosuccinate

WHEN TO USE SULFATE-CONTAINING SHAMPOOS

There is definitely a role for the occasional use of sulfate containing shampoos. Remember, these shampoos do the best job at cleansing the hair. Many companies are starting to label sulfate containing shampoos as "clarifying" shampoos just to emphasize the level of cleanliness that is achieved after using them.

For my patients who prefer to wash only with conditioner (see Chapter 8), I recommend the use of a sulfate containing shampoo at least once a month. These shampoos are also helpful after removing braided or weaved styles that have been in place for several weeks. Many of my patients find it difficult to wash their hair on a regular basis when they are wearing extensions and when the extensions are removed there is usually weeks of buildup underneath. If you have straight hair and find that a sulfate-free shampoo is not cleaning your hair well enough, try a shampoo with a sulfate that is lower down on the sulfate list so that you minimize the effects of drying the hair. After shampooing you should always follow with a rich conditioner to counteract the drying effects of the shampoo.

Five

Look for These Ingredients in Your Shampoo

So now that you've figured out that your sulfate-containing shampoo is working against you, what should you do next? Shopping for new hair products can be exhausting, and you will truly have to prepare for trial and error. To get you started, I've identified two ingredients that you can look for, in your shampoos.

GENTLE SHAMPOO INGREDIENTS TO BE ON THE LOOKOUT FOR

1. Decyl Glucoside: While sulfate containing ingredients come with a negative charge that can leave your hair feeling frizzy, decyl glucoside is in a class of ingredients called *non-ionic surfactants*. These shampoo ingredients have no charge at all, meaning they are less likely to leave your hair feeling dry. They work well with other shampoo ingredients and for that reason is a common ingredient in many popular shampoos. Decyl glucoside is one of the most common ingredients that you will find in a sulfate-free shampoo in the market, and for good reason.

2. Cocamidopropyl Betaine: This is another common ingredient found in sulfate free shampoos. Unlike decyl glucoside, it actually carries two charges, a positive and a negative one, which cancel each other out to leave a neutral charge on the hair. This means

that it is referred to as an *amphoteric surfactant*. As a result, shampoos with this ingredient tend to do less damage to the hair. Some people are sensitive to this ingredient so while it works really well, if you have a known sensitivity to it, be sure to steer clear.

There is also one ingredient that you should be aware of because it looks like it is a harsh ingredient, when in fact it is a gentle cleansing agent:

3. <u>Behentrimonium methosulfate</u>: Even though it has sulfate at the end of its name, behentrimonium methosulfate is not an anionic surfactant (it's actually a positively charged *cationic surfactant*) and is totally safe to use regularly.

These ingredients are less likely to strip your hair of protective oils and, in the long run, can help minimize breakage. When looking for a new shampoo with one or both of these ingredients, you want to make sure it's near the top of the ingredients list. That is a sign that it's doing most of the heavy lifting in the shampoo. If it's toward the end of the ingredients list, it likely means that only a tiny amount of it is in the shampoo and it's not playing as much of a role.

Below is a list of other gentle ingredients you may find in your shampoos.

Gentle Cleansing Ingredients
Benzalkonium Chloride
Cetrimonium Chloride
Cocamidopropyl Betaine
Decyl Glucoside
Lauryl Glucoside
Stearamidopropyl Dimethylamine
Cocamide MEA
Disodium Cocoamphodipropionate
Behentrimonium Methosulfate

Six

Apply Oil to Your Hair
Before Washing

I know what you're thinking: why on earth would I apply oil to my hair before I shampoo if the whole point is to clean it?

As I mentioned in Chapter 3, shampooing the hair is a necessary evil. When sebum, the natural protective oil produced by the scalp, coats the hair strands, it attracts dirt. Hair products, like gels, mousses, and conditioners do the same thing. Over time, this dirt and grease build up and require a proper cleansing to get rid of the film. This is where shampooing comes in. But the mere act of washing the hair is dangerous in and of itself.

When water hits your strands, it causes immediate swelling of your hair. The scientific name for this process is "hygral fatigue." If your hair is weakened for whatever reason, rapid swelling can lead to sudden breakage as well as tangling of your hair. One effective way to combat this process is to apply an oil to your hair immediately BEFORE you shampoo.

If you want to get your hair squeaky clean, then maybe you want to skip this step, especially if your hair is really dirty and you're okay losing a couple of extra strands. If your hair is not too dirty and you're finding yourself in a period of excessive hair breakage, then this is an easy step to include in your wash day routine.

When it comes to research, coconut oil is the only oil that's been shown to prevent hygral fatigue but it is likely that many oils work just as well. This is because the particles that make up coconut oil are small enough to penetrate into the hair shaft. Avoid thick, viscous oils like castor oil as chances are you won't be able to wash this away cleanly. Consider oils like grape seed, jojoba, and olive oil instead if you prefer to avoid coconut oil. Try it during your next wash and consider making it a permanent addition to your routine if you like what you see!

Seven

Make Sure to Keep Your Dandruff Under Control

In the quest for healthy hair, dandruff can be quite the annoying foe. Most people are familiar with the type of dandruff that leads to annoying small flakes on your favorite shirt, but dandruff can be much worse than that. Many people have dandruff that leads not only to thick flaking but hair loss and bleeding on the scalp; we dermatologists call this seborrheic dermatitis. In these instances, it is best to see a dermatologist for prescription treatment.

So what if you fall somewhere in the middle and you think your dandruff is keeping you from having healthy locks? Here are a few suggestions:

1. Consider slightly increasing how often you shampoo your hair. For instance, if you wash your hair three times a week, consider going up to five times a week. If you shampoo your hair once a week, consider upping to twice a week. Washing the hair more often actually can help keep dandruff under control. You should only follow this recommendation if you...

2. Use a sulfate-free dandruff shampoo. This task is much easier said than done. Most dandruff shampoos are formulated with sulfates to increase cleansing power, which as I mentioned, helps control dandruff. However, if you are going to increase how often you shampoo, it will be important that you find a sulfate free dandruff

shampoo so that you do not damage your hair in the process. You can alternate between a normal dandruff shampoo and a sulfate free shampoo if you find that the sulfate free shampoo is not doing the job.

3. Don't convince yourself that dandruff is just a sign that your scalp is dry. While it is true that scaly skin is often dry skin, the same is not true for the scalp. Dandruff is actually caused by a commonly found yeast called *Malassezia*, that probably lives on all of us and dandruff is a sign of our body's unique response to this yeast. However, only some of us will develop dandruff even with the same amounts of yeast on the scalp. All of this is to say, it is not enough to simply apply oil to the scalp in hopes of getting rid of dandruff, you must treat the cause. In the long run, it will do wonders for your hair.

4. Be patient. There is no cure for dandruff, so you will have to be prepared to treat it for the long run.

Eight

Condition Your Hair Every Time You Wash (With or Without Shampoo!)

As I have mentioned several times before (because it is so important!), our scalp produces a natural moisturizer, called sebum, that helps protect our hair strands. In fact, for those with tightly curled hair, it is essential to replace the action of sebum through the use of a daily conditioner.

You can think of conditioners as synthetic sebum, as they are literally designed to mimic the action of sebum on the hair strand. So if your hair is not getting naturally coated by sebum, then manually applying it to the hair will do wonders.

Not only will a conditioner protect your hair, but it also helps to balance out the negative charge left behind by shampoos and prevents hair breakage. By balancing out the negative charge left behind by shampoos, conditioners help to leave the hair soft and shiny. Conditioners can also temporarily mend split ends by bringing together two layers of your hair shaft. Aren't they just magical?

While conditioning the hair after shampooing is a must, more frequent use can be helpful for those with really dry hair, especially curly or damaged hair.

One way to pack more conditioning into your hair care routine is to wash your hair with conditioner alone. Conditioners actually have mild cleansing ability, so if your hair is not too dirty, this is a reasonable option, but this won't work for everyone. If your hair gets greasy quickly, you will definitely not want to wash with conditioner alone; in this case, opting for a gentle shampoo makes more sense.

If you want to play around with washing your hair with a conditioner alone and skipping shampooing, start slow. I usually recommend two conditioner-only wash sessions for every one shampoo + conditioner cleansing session for my patients with dry or damaged hair.

Some shampoos are branded as "co-wash" shampoos; this means that they are formulated more like a conditioner, and can be used in place of a standard rinse out conditioner for this intended use. Over time, however, overuse of conditioners can lead to buildup (remember, they attract dirt, just like sebum) and eventually shampooing is needed to get your hair clean. For women who choose to add conditioner-only washing sessions to their regimen, the occasional use of sulfate containing shampoos is necessary to help rid the hair of buildup. Additionally, I do not recommend washing with conditioner only before a deep conditioning or protein treatment session because these will likely be less effective.

Nine

Look for These Ingredients in Your Conditioner

C onditioners are awesome, and I hope by now I have convinced you of that fact. So what should you look for in a conditioner?

HIGH-YIELD CONDITIONER INGREDIENTS

1. Stearyl alcohol or cetyl alcohol: even though you see the word alcohol, these ingredients help to soften the hair. They also help minimize friction in your hair so that your hair is less likely to tangle and split. If you like your hair to feel soft and smooth after you wash, then check your conditioner for these ingredients

2. Dimethicone: this is a type of silicone which helps the hair feel smooth and look shiny after use. Dimethicone is commonly found in smoothing serums, leave in, and rinse out conditioners because of these very properties. Some people choose to avoid silicones because they can leave a thin film on the hair that can be undesirable.

3. Hydrolyzed keratin/collagen/elastin etc.: When you see these ingredients in a conditioner, it means that it has protein in it which can add additional strength to your hair. However, sometimes protein can make the hair feel a little drier, even if it does seem stronger. If you prefer that your hair feel as soft as possible, then

you should avoid these ingredients in your conditioner except for when you are specifically doing protein treatments. Protein treatments often have higher amounts of these ingredients than protein-containing conditioners.

4. Citric acid, benzoic acid, glutamic acid, etc.: these acids help leave a positive charge on the hair which reduces flyaways and frizz. These are great ingredients to look for if you are looking for your hair to be more manageable and shiny.

There are many other ingredients that can make a conditioner perfect for you so don't be dismayed if your favorite conditioner is missing these ingredients. However, if you are new to your healthy hair journey and don't know where to start, use this list as a guide to help you navigate the ever dreaded beauty aisle.

Ten

Deep Condition Your Hair Regularly

Hair that has been damaged by bleaching, relaxing, hair coloring or by any other method is often dry and brittle. It has a more difficult time holding onto and retaining moisture that either comes naturally from the scalp or in the form of a conditioner. For people with healthy, minimally damaged hair, a simple washing regimen consisting of shampoo + conditioner probably works just fine. However, if you're reading this book because you're a) experiencing difficulties getting it to grow long or you're b) noticing more breakage, then that regimen is simply not enough.

Enter the role of deep conditioners. These are more intensive conditioners that are designed to stay on the hair for extended periods of time. They are often intended to be used with heat, which allows the scales of the hair cuticle (think of them like shingles on a roof) to lift up so that the conditioner can penetrate more deeply. So while the benefits of a regular conditioner may last a couple of days, the benefits of a deep conditioning treatment can last for a week or longer. Regular use of a deep conditioner helps mend split ends temporarily and provide more resistance to breakage from daily grooming. You can mix your deep conditioners with oils to provide an even more intensive moisturizing experience.

I typically recommend adjusting how often you deep condition based on your hair type or hair condition:

- Healthy naturally curly/kinky hair- deep condition at least once weekly.
- Damaged naturally curly/kinky hair-deep condition twice weekly for a few months if you are new to moisturizing your hair and your hair is in need of TLC. Add a protein treatment once weekly during this time
- Healthy naturally straight/wavy- deep condition once monthly
- Damaged naturally straight/wavy hair-alternate deep conditioning and protein treatments every other week for three months until health is restored

Eleven

Use a Leave-In Conditioner

Applying a conditioner to your hair is like doing the job your scalp is supposed to do when sebum is not cutting it. Leave in conditioners do the job of keeping your hair moisturized in between washes. For most curly haired girls (and others with really dry hair), adding a leave-in conditioner to your regimen is an absolute must. Because there are definite downsides to washing the hair every day, if you have dry, damaged hair, you will need to find another way to add moisture back in. This is where a leave-in conditioner comes in.

Leave-in conditioners contain some of the same ingredients that are found in regular conditioners but are not meant to be washed out and are generally lightweight, so they do not weigh your hair down. There are water-based leave-ins (for those who require only minimal mid-week moisture) and cream-based leave-in conditioners as well. Remember, you are looking for something that will mimic the action of sebum on the hair, so using products like serums and glossers may make your hair feel smooth, but they are not truly conditioning the hair.

If your hair is on the drier side and you would like to incorporate leave-in conditioners, then I recommend the following based on your hair type:

- Straight or wavy hair (color or heat damaged in particular)- apply water-based leave-in conditioner immediately after shampooing and conditioning to wet hair. If you are shampooing 3–5×/week, then no additional use is necessary during the week

- Curly/Kinky chemical-free/natural hair: apply water or cream based leave-in conditioner after shampooing and conditioning 5–7× during the week. Choose your leave-in conditioner based on the density of your hair. Follow with an oil to trap moisture in the hair

When applying, make sure to drench the ends of your hair in conditioner as this is the part of your hair that is least likely to be coated with protective sebum. Your leave-in conditioner should leave your hair feeling softer, and you should immediately notice less breakage from styling. If this is not the result you are getting from your leave-in, keep searching until you are satisfied.

Twelve

Apply Conditioner to Your Hair Before Swimming

Swimming is a fantastic activity to engage in; it's relaxing and provides an excellent cardiovascular workout. However, the chlorine in pools can be incredibly damaging and more drying than even the worst sulfate containing shampoo. This is one of the reasons that women with really curly or kinky hair rightly shy away from swimming regularly. The adverse effects of swimming can be minimized by washing the chlorine out of the hair immediately after leaving the pool though this may not be enough if water alone dries your hair.

If you (or your child) has dry or damaged hair and are planning to hit the pool soon, consider the following routine to minimize damage during your next pool visit:

1. Apply a thick conditioner to your hair before entering the pool. Leave in conditioners work but definitely do not protect as well as a rinse out or deep conditioner. Obviously, you do not want to apply something that will create a lot of suds in the pool, so play around with different products beforehand. The closer to pool time that you apply it, the better off you will be. A thick, hair grease can be applied as an alternative as this will prevent any water and damaging chemicals from penetrating your hair but will not necessarily keep your hair moisturized. You will also likely

require a clarifying shampoo to wash the petrolatum out of your hair.

2. Rinse your hair after you exit the pool; this will get as much chlorine out of your hair as possible.
3. Plan on shampooing and deep conditioning your hair either the same day or the next day to help replenish the moisture that your hair has lost in the pool.

With these tips in hand, you no longer have to worry about your hair getting in the way of a good time!

Thirteen

Add Regular Protein Treatments to Your Regimen

Almost anyone reading this book will benefit from incorporating protein treatments into their regimen, some more than others. Protein treatments and protein-containing conditioners are marketed toward people with damaged hair and often use the words "repairing" or "reconstructing" in the title. As I am sure you are aware, our hair is made of protein, specifically keratin. Over time, harsh styling habits break down keratin leaving the hair susceptible to breakage. If you were able to look at a strand of hair under a special microscope, you would actually be able to visualize small holes dotted throughout the hair, and the more holes present along the hair, the weaker it is.

Enter protein treatments. These products contain small, or hydrolyzed, proteins that are small enough to enter the hair shaft and temporarily fill in these gaps. This results in hair that is stronger and can also lead to the appearance of fuller hair. The great thing is, the more damaged your hair is, the better they work! That's because if there are more holes to fill in, the more noticeable the results will be.

Protein treatments should be applied with heat, which lifts up the outer portion of the hair allowing protein treatments to penetrate more deeply into the hair.

How often you use protein treatments depends on the extent of your hair damage. For hair that's been severely damaged, protein treatments once weekly for at least 1–3 months is ideal. However, most women can likely get away with using protein treatments once every few months. Women with thin hair will benefit from using protein treatments more frequently. This is because they are often missing an elusive third layer of the hair shaft, called the medulla, which means damage to the innermost portion of the hair shaft is more likely. Personally, I try to make sure I do a light protein treatment on my hair every week.

One potential downside to protein treatments is that they can occasionally make the hair feel dry and straw-like. If this is true for you, then you will need to follow with a deep conditioner or a really rich moisturizing conditioner after every use. The benefits of a protein treatment only last until the next shampoo, but with regular use, you will experience less breakage which will allow your hair to grow thicker and longer. Who wouldn't love that?

Fourteen

Search Google or YouTube for Help

It's not often that you hear a doctor refer patients to Google for help. While googling medical conditions can send you into a downward spiral of inaccurate self-diagnoses, googling hairstyling tips can be quite helpful for those who are newbies when it comes to styling their own hair.

There is one unspoken rule to achieving healthy hair, and that is getting to know your hair inside and out. Most of us cannot afford to have a stylist take care of our hair on a weekly, much less daily, basis so part of your new hair care journey will have to involve getting up close and personal with your hair.

For many who will read this book, this will seem intuitive, but the truth is, many of my clients have spent most of their lives doing minimal hair care in between stylist appointments. This means that when issues arise- such as breakage, thinning, or difficulty growing hair to long lengths, these women are at a loss about what to do. That is what eventually leads them to my office.

During these appointments, I do what I have done in this book- I give them a long list of hair tips and products that they should abide by to improve the health of their hair. When I get the deer-in-headlights look at terms like "weekly deep-conditioning" and "bi-weekly protein-treatments" that is when I know that a little more guidance is needed.

The great thing about Google, and in particular YouTube, is that you can find a video on almost anything. If the beauty aisle is too daunting and you need to get a deep conditioner recommendation, you can find someone with similar hair giving a detailed review on your product of interest. If you need to figure out how to style your hair for a special event, there's undoubtedly someone on YouTube who can walk you through that too.

Of course, everything you find online has to be taken with a grain of salt. Many of the most prominent YouTubers are paid to endorse hair and makeup products so this may lead to biased reviews of hair products. Influencers, the name given to men and women who get paid to use their social media pages to sell products, can make tens to hundreds of thousands of dollars by making videos like these, so the incentive to be biased is real.

When approached correctly, Google and YouTube can be powerful tools which provide a wealth of resources. It is so very important for every woman to feel comfortable taking care of her own hair. For many women, there is almost no way to achieve healthy hair without taking this step. It is of particular importance to curly-haired women who will need to apply a conditioner every day to prevent breakage. If nothing else, I want women to walk away from this book feeling empowered with understanding that they control their own (hair) destiny.

Fifteen

Reconsider Potentially Harmful Ingredients

Have you ever wondered who polices the safety of your cosmetic products? What most people do not know is that, ingredients in non-prescription cosmetic products sold in the United States, are not tightly regulated by the Food and Drug Administration (FDA). This is in contrast to the European Union, which actually does a good job keeping a close eye on the products their citizens are using. In the United States, harmful ingredients must be brought to the attention of the FDA by consumers like you and me. If there are enough complaints, then the FDA may politely ask companies to avoid using these ingredients in their products, but more likely than not, they will not check to see if the ingredients are removed. It is only on the rare occasion that the FDA will actually ban an ingredient. However, even this is tough to enforce. This is because when a company provides an ingredients list on the label, the only code they are following is the honor system. In other terms, this means that companies can choose to be open about all the ingredients or they could leave them off altogether.

While I do believe that the vast majority of ingredients found in cosmetic products are absolutely safe, I will use this chapter to shed light on some of the ingredients that have been associated with some controversy. Unlike the ingredients I have discussed in other chapters, these ingredients are not necessarily harmful to your hair, but are controversial because of potential side effects they may have on your body.

CONTROVERSIAL PRODUCT INGREDIENTS

1. Methylisothiazolinone (MIT): though this ingredient is banned in Europe, it is a common ingredient found in many shampoos and conditioners sold in the United States. It is popular among manufacturers because it helps extend the shelf life of the products, so they don't expire or spoil too quickly. Despite this upside, they are also a common cause of allergic reactions. Not sure if you are allergic to MIT? If you find that your scalp starts itching every time you wash it, check your label to see if this is the culprit and opt for an MIT-free alternative.

2. Parabens: Like MIT, parabens are common ingredients used to extend the shelf- life of many cosmetic items and foods. Parabens are controversial because of their hormone-like activity. In animal studies, parabens have been shown to act very similarly to estrogen on the body BUT are much weaker than normal estrogen (like 10,000–100,000 times weaker). In these studies, animals are exposed to very large doses of parabens, much larger than the doses we find our products. It is unclear if this has any significant impact in terms of diseases and the human body gets rid of parabens within an hour on average. So far, there is no evidence of any negative effect on the body, but more and more companies have started removing them from their products to be on the safe side. You can tell if your product has parabens by merely looking for the word in your ingredients list (like methylparaben, ethylparaben, etc.)

3. Phthalates- This is a sneaky one because you will rarely see phthalates plainly listed on an ingredients label. Instead, they are usually listed simply as "fragrance." In some studies on mice, phthalates were shown to lower testosterone levels in the body, but

like parabens, the overall impact on the human body is unclear. Phthalates are also being used less frequently because of heightened awareness by consumers.

4. Sodium Lauryl Sulfate- I have already discussed the drying effects of SLS in this book, but you should also be aware that this ingredient is a common cause of skin irritation. People suffering from dandruff are more likely to react to this ingredient. If you've tried avoiding MIT and you still notice an itchy scalp that gets worse after shampooing, then make sure you look for a shampoo that is SLS free.

It is important to do your research on any product you use. You may find that you have been using products with these ingredients for years with no issues. If you prefer to be on the safe side, many products do not contain these ingredients and can work just as well for your hair.

Sixteen

Avoid Chemical Styling Treatments

If there's one thing I have learned as a hair loss specialist, it's that everyone (including me, sometimes!) wants what they can't have. My curly haired patients do everything in their power to get their hair straight and lament the fact that their hair is so difficult to "control." My straight haired patients want hair with more "body." Brunettes want to be blonde, and blondes want to be redheads. And the beauty industry is right there to satisfy all of our greatest dreams and desires for our hair. However, there is a big downside to permanently altering the appearance of our hair, and that is the strength of the hair.

Let's start with the basics. If you were to break down the chemical composition of the hair, you would see that it is made up of strong bonds, called disulfide bonds, and weak bonds, called hydrogen bonds. Any permanent styling treatment, whether it is relaxing the hair or dying it, first works by breaking the disulfide bonds. To do this, the hair has to be exposed to an agent strong enough (usually one with a high pH value) that can break the bond. Once broken, those bonds are never the same again and do not provide the same strength they were once able to provide. Breaking these sulfide bonds leads to more holes within the hair shaft which is one of the reasons why protein treatments are a must.

Before you rack your brain trying to figure out if your bleach blonde hair can be full and healthy, ask yourself if you really need it to be bleached blonde. If your goal in reading this book is to have your healthiest hair ever, then you'll have to closely examine just how badly you want that dye job or relaxer treatment. You may find that by altering other parts of your regimen you can still have hair you love, and while it may not be the hair of your dreams, you can come pretty close. For instance, if you decide to dye your hair blonde, be prepared to add in a weekly deep conditioning to combat the dryness created by coloring your hair. Or, if you prefer to have your hair relaxed, you should plan to commit to regular protein treatments.

GOING NATURAL

What does it mean to 'go natural'? For women with curly hair who have spent years relaxing their hair straight, it means embracing your natural curl pattern and giving your hair the best opportunity to thrive. For many women, this is a dramatic paradigm shift, and there is a lot of fear associated with allowing the world to see a side of you that has been hidden for many years. Consider a woman in her late 20's or early 30's who has very little idea about what her hair naturally looks like because she started straightening her hair before she formed memories (I may or may not be talking about myself here).

If you are trying to figure out what your hair will look like once it is curly, it's helpful to get an understanding of your "curl type." One widely accepted hair typing system divides hair into four types 1: straight 2: wavy 3: curly and 4: coily. Each type is divided into three subtypes: A, B, and C, each with increasing levels of curl. Compared to straight hair of the same length and density, curly hair appears more full and is great option for people with thinning or fine hair. If you have naturally very curly hair and specifically tightly coiled hair (think type 4B/4C) then these are some things for you to keep in mind about going natural:

1. Be prepared to give your hair extra TLC; compared to straight hair, going natural does not require less hair upkeep, it requires more.

Don't be fooled into thinking that once you stop relaxing your hair it will suddenly become thick and full. Remember, curly hair is more fragile because it has more difficulty holding onto moisture, and each twist and turn of a curl is an inherent point of weakness. This means that you will need to dedicate the time needed to deep condition and leave in condition regularly, to counteract the natural characteristics of curly hair. When treated right, naturally curly hair can reflect a beauty like none other, but when treated poorly it can leave you feeling very disappointed.

2. You can't be natural in name only; you must learn to embrace your natural curl. I can't tell you how many women I have met who have come to me complaining about hair breakage and don't understand why their hair is not growing even though they stopped relaxing their hair. Usually, these women still wear their hair straight and do this by flat ironing their hair every day. This absolutely defeats the purpose. I would argue that flat ironing the hair daily does MORE damage to the hair than a relaxer, though I will explain more about this, later. If you have curly hair and you're going natural, you must let go of the idea of having straight hair on a regular basis.

3. Figure out a natural style that you feel comfortable wearing daily. Before you go natural you should come up with a game plan. Scour social media websites for examples of women with natural hair and identify hairstyles that you feel comfortable wearing. If your hair is less tightly curled (like 2C-3C), you may find that your natural hair is amenable to styles that require little more than conditioner and a styling gel (a wash n' go style). This cuts down some of your maintenance time. Buns, braids and twisted styles are good options to wear during the week for curlier hair types.

4. Avoid hiding your natural hair under wigs and weaves. Again, if your goal is to have healthier, longer, stronger hair and your hair is naturally curly, it is going to require regular upkeep and TLC. If your hair is always covered by a weave, it is nearly impossible to

condition it as often as is necessary. While wigs and weaves can be great to protect the hair from the ravages of daily grooming, they should be used in moderation only.

If all of this sounds reasonable and you're ready to cut out chemical styling, good for you! You are that much closer to healthier hair. If you've read this and have determined that giving up relaxers are not for you, then keep reading for tips on how to maximize the health of your hair in spite of chemical treatments and learn about healthy alternatives.

Seventeen

Consider Firing Your Stylist

A stylist is like a best friend, a therapist and a doctor all rolled up in one. For many people, they are not just a stylist, they are family. Which is why what I am about to say will be hard to hear: Fire your stylist. Or at least think seriously about whether you should get a new one.

Stylists can be amazing; they offer hand-holding and can teach you how to take care of your hair properly. They also have access to products that frankly are not available to the general public which can result in beautiful results that you just can't seem to achieve at home. A great stylist can do what few can: keep your hair looking great and healthy, but in reality, great stylists are limited.

If you are loyal to your stylist and are dealing with recurrent hair breakage and thinning, then your stylist may be part of the problem. Not on purpose of course, but you know what they say about good intentions. Most stylists want to make their clients look their best, but this may come at the cost of the health of their hair. Not sure if you should be on the hunt for a new stylist? Answer a few questions below:

1. On balance, does your stylist discuss ways to camouflage your thinning hair (weaves, clip-ins, updos) instead of discussing methods to improve it?
2. Does your stylist continue to perform harmful styling habits (flat iron multiple times, use bleaching agents, leave the relaxer on for

longer than necessary) even when you repeatedly ask them to stop?

3. Does your stylist ignore you when you say you are experiencing pain from a styling treatment (e.g., burning from relaxer treatment or during flat ironing, tight extensions, etc.)?

4. When you ask for tips on taking care of your hair at home (including tips on how to do routine hair care that is also available at the salon), does your stylist refuse to teach you and insist you continue to receive all your hair care from them?

5. When you experience a bad outcome from a harmful styling treatment, does the stylist try and deflect all blame back onto you?

6. Does your stylist regularly exceed recommended application times for permanent styling treatments such as chemical straightening and hair coloring?

If you answered yes to two or more of these questions, then you may need a new stylist. Consider asking friends for recommendations and try out new stylists for minor services such as a wash and blow dry. You'll likely be able to tell after one treatment if the stylist is one who thinks critically about hair. A great stylist prioritizes the long term health of your hair over the short term appearance. If you are not educated about what healthy hair practices are, a lousy stylist may convince you that harmful styling habits are actually *good* for you. Your stylist also shouldn't be afraid to tell you no when you insist on bleach blonde color that is certain to worsen your hair's damage.

It is not uncommon for my patients with hair loss to report back that their stylist was unwilling to adjust their hair care regimen to improve their hair's health. Hairstyling should not be a one size fits all. A stylist should be able to do an assessment and tailor your hair care specifically to you, just as a doctor would. The stylist-client relationship is truly a partnership and one that pays off dividends when done right.

Eighteen

Reconsider Dyeing Your Hair

I see patients of all races and ages and without fail the styling habit that patients are most resistant to giving up is dyeing their hair. By the time patients come to my office, they have been dyeing their hair a specific color for years, for some, even decades. Our hair is such an integral part of who we are and how we see ourselves. Some of us see ourselves as blondes even though we were born brunettes.

You have already heard my position on permanent styling treatments, they damage the hair, and there is really no way to avoid that. However, there are many different ways to color the hair, some of which may be more damaging than others.

Hair dyes work by opening up the hair shaft so that color can be deposited as close to the cortex, (the inner part of your hair shaft,) as possible. This is the part of your hair responsible for its strength. There are many chemical reactions involved in this process but to simplify it, the closer to the core the hair color gets, the longer it sticks around and the more damage it does in order to get there.

The pigment responsible for dark hair is very stubborn (red pigment is even more stubborn) so it is much easier to work with the pigment and make hair darker than it is to completely remove the pigment and make the hair lighter. So, if your goal is to get hair color that lasts then damage is unavoidable. Even semi-permanent dye requires hydrogen peroxide to open up the hair cuticle so that the dyeing process can occur.

To dye the hair a lighter color, it must first be bleached with hydrogen peroxide, giving the hair a yellow or orange color, a result of permanently wiping away the pigment of the hair. Afterward, a dye of any color is applied to the hair to give it its final appearance. Depending on the desired final appearance, higher or lower concentrations of hydrogen peroxide (referred to as the *volume*) are used. So for example, if you have naturally brown hair and just want to dye your hair light brown, only a low concentration of a bleaching agent is needed. But if your hair is naturally almost black and you want to become blonde, nearly 100 percent of your natural pigment will need to be stripped away, thus requiring a high concentration bleaching agent.

Unfortunately, hydrogen peroxide strips away keratin and leaves the hair weaker than when it started. Over time this process adds up leaving the hair more prone to breakage. The loss in protein can be drastic, especially when the hair is bleached, and is one of the reasons why dyed hair can feel so dry and brittle all the time. It's tough to have healthy, vibrant hair that's been permanently dyed.

Hair dyes also often contain an ingredient called paraphenylenediamine, or PPD for short. This is an ingredient that is useful for dyeing the hair darker colors and can even be found in temporary rinses. It is one of the most common causes of allergic reactions, and the reaction can be severe. A quick Google search of allergic reactions to hair dye will pull up dozens of images of men and women with red face and eyes swollen shut. Treatment usually requires at least a short course of steroids by mouth. I know what you're thinking: "Why not just avoid hair dyes with PPD?" Trust me, this is much easier said than done. Even natural hair dyes are often combined with PPD for a more drastic effect. There are, however, a select group of hair dyes that are PPD free (such as Goldwell's Elumen brand) that can provide long-lasting bright colors to the hair but may not provide the full range of more natural colors that traditional dyes can provide.

TYPES OF HAIR DYE

1. Temporary hair dye or rinses: This type of hair color is the least likely to cause hair damage because they are designed to last a maximum of one or two shampooings. The hair color actually physically sits on top of the hair and does not get close to the core of the hair shaft at all. Unfortunately, temporary hair dyes cannot lighten the hair, they only make it darker and they do a bad job of covering gray hair.

2. Semi or Demi-Permanent dyes: These hair dyes are designed to last anywhere between 6 and 12 shampoos (fewer if you are using a harsh sulfate-containing shampoo). These dyes use hydrogen peroxide to get a little bit closer to the core of the hair shaft. However, because the dye does not quite reach the core of the hair shaft, it will not work well to lighten the hair, but only darken it.

3. Permanent Hair Dyes: permanent synthetic dyes are the most commonly used dyes because they last the longest and can be used to dye the hair any color, light or dark. They often contain hydrogen peroxide at higher levels (20–40 vol. solutions) than semi-permanent dyes. Unlike semi and demi-permanent dyes, most permanent hair dyes also contain ammonia, which allows hair color to reach the cortex of the hair. Some permanent dyes are labeled as "ammonia-free" but contain an ingredient, ethanolamine, that works in a similar way. Ammonia-free permanent dyes should not be considered to be any less damaging to the hair than ammonia-containing dyes, so don't let fancy marketing fool you.

If all of that is hard to remember, this table provides a quick summary of differences:

	PPD?	Ammonia or Ethanolamine?	Hydrogen Peroxide?	Lighten the hair?	Cover Grays?	Durability	Hair Damage
Rinses	Yes	No	No	No	No	1–2 Shampoos	Low
Semi-Permanent	Yes	No	Yes	No	Yes	6–8 Shampoos	Moderate
Demi-Permanent	Yes	No	Yes	No	Yes	10–12 Shampoos	Moderate
Permanent Hair Dye Including Bleaching	Yes	Yes	Yes	Yes	Yes	Permanent	High

So what's a girl to do if she loves hair color and is tired of the damage? Here are a few hair coloring tips:

1. Avoid lightening your hair if possible. Coloring your hair a darker color with a semi or demi-permanent hair dye will do less damage than lightening it (or darkening it) with a permanent hair color.
2. If you are looking to lighten your hair, ask your stylist to apply the lowest concentration of hydrogen peroxide possible to achieve your final hair color. If they have been applying 30 vol. in the past, ask them to try a 20 vol. bleaching solution before applying the hair color. Of course, the final color will be different, but you can be spared some damage.
3. Never perform two chemical treatments on the same day. Getting a chemical relaxer or perm on the same day as your color appointment can cause permanent damage, and at worst, hair falling out in clumps.
4. Deep condition the hair, after you have colored your hair and incorporate weekly protein treatments to your regimen, to help restore the protein loss that has occurred.
5. Consider natural alternatives to hair dye, like henna, to cover your grays instead of synthetic dyes.

Nineteen

Use a Lye Relaxer Only

For many faithful users of relaxer, the relationship with relaxer begins at a young age. I can attest to that because I also had my first relaxer at a very young age. I remember getting very frustrated when my "new growth" started to arrive because it meant it was time for a new relaxer.

People often assume that because I am a dermatologist specializing in hair loss, I am an enemy of chemical relaxers. Many of my patients who relax their hair will start their appointments defiantly proclaiming that they refuse to stop relaxing their hair because that is what they are used to dermatologists telling them to do. So, let me start out by saying this:

I am not an enemy of chemical relaxers, but my goal is to make my patients knowledgeable about the side effects.

I am not an enemy of relaxers because I know there are several pros associated with the use of relaxer, such as:

- Ease of styling (this is huge and can mean the difference between minutes in the mirror vs. hours!)
- Permanent straightening for those who like to wear their hair straight most of the time
- General personal preference

Of course, as a hair loss specialist, these days I concern myself more with the cons of relaxers as I think it is prudent for each person to balance the pros and cons in their life before proceeding. These include:

- Chemical burns
- Weak, limp hair
- Temporary or Permanent hair loss
- Recurrent Hair Breakage

So let's start with the basics.

WHAT IS A CHEMICAL RELAXER?

Chemical relaxers are most commonly divided into lye and no-lye formulations. Lye formulations are typically available only in salons and contain sodium hydroxide. No-lye formulations, on the other hand, are available over the counter and often have to be mixed before use. The most popular formulations contain calcium hydroxide (base) and guanidine carbonate (activator), which when mixed together form guanidine hydroxide.

If you recall from your high school chemistry class, pH scales run from 1 to 14, with numbers below 7 representing acids and number above 7 representing bases. The extremes of the pH scales contain ingredients that can easily burn through skin, plastic and even metal depending on the concentration. Lye formulations typically measure at a pH of 11–13 (!), and no-lye formulations typically measure at a pH of 9–11. This is why people generally associate lye relaxers with more severe burns than no-lye formulations.

SO WHY ARE LYE RELAXERS BETTER THAN NO-LYE RELAXERS?

I know this sounds crazy. For women like me who have been familiar with relaxer their whole lives, no-lye relaxer is considered the safe version of relaxer because it takes longer to burn the scalp. They are readily available over the counter because no company wants to be sued for causing a severe burn to the scalp. That's the one upside of a no-lye relaxer but other than that, it's all downside.

For starters: remember how I said no-lye relaxers are made of calcium hydroxide? Well, that's what's found in limewater. When it's mixed with guanidine carbonate, calcium carbonate is formed as a by-product, and that's also known as limestone. While these ingredients are effective at relaxing the hair, these calcified deposits build up on the hair over time causing it to become dull and more susceptible to damage. That dullness is one of the reasons why hair that's relaxed at home does not look quite as shiny as hair that has been consistently relaxed at a salon.

But there is another reason I prefer salon relaxers: the burn. You read that right. While I never advise that relaxer is kept on the hair until the scalp burns, the mere fear of burning the scalp because of the caustic characteristics of lye relaxer means that it is rarely left on longer than instructed. This is different than home relaxers, which users frequently leave on for much longer than instructed in hopes of getting hair that is "bone straight." Instead of relying on a timer to estimate when the processing of the hair is complete, a tingling and/or a mild burning sensation is often considered a more reliable metric that women use to inform them of when to rinse relaxer from the hair. Burning and tingling sensations are a sign that the skin is getting irritated, not that the relaxer is working. I will say that again in case it is not clear:

Burning and tingling is a sign that the skin is getting irritated
(i.e., burned), not that the relaxer is working.

Because no-lye relaxers are designed to lessen skin irritation, they are often left on longer than lye containing relaxer formulations. This means that women are much more likely to over-process the hair using no-lye relaxer kits. This is what leads to more breakage, more dulling and generally, more problems.

The decision to relax the hair should never be taken lightly. It is a permanent, irreversible treatment that works by first weakening your hair strands. If you desire to have hair that is thick and dense, relaxer will likely do the opposite. However, it is a wiser alternative than using extreme heat every week to straighten the hair.

If you have decided that, even after knowing this, you would like to keep relaxing your hair, here are some helpful tips to minimize damage:

1. If you want to truly just "relax" your curls, and not get it bone straight, consider asking your stylist to apply relaxers with a lower concentration of sodium hydroxide. These relaxers are typically marketed to kids or have the words "mild" on the box. Some people call this a texturizer, which is just a low concentration relaxer. While this will not eliminate the damage experienced from using a relaxer, it should minimize it.
2. Use a lye relaxer only and make sure it is applied by a stylist
3. Always make sure to use a neutralizing shampoo, NOT a regular shampoo, when rinsing relaxer from the hair.
4. Get a hydrating or deep conditioner treatment applied the same day as your relaxer to help add moisture
5. Apply a protein treatment to your hair weekly (but not on the day of your relaxer) to prevent further breakage
6. Deep condition your hair every time you wash
7. Eliminate or limit the use of heat styling tools to straighten your hair

Twenty

Space Out Chemical Styling Treatments

The great thing about hair is that it's always growing. But sometimes the worst thing about hair is that's always growing, ugh! This is an issue when you're an avid fan of permanent styling treatments like relaxers and hair coloring. That's because, every few weeks, like clockwork, you realize that you're due for another treatment.

Let's say you've read my chapters on how harmful these treatments can be, but you've determined that cutting them out completely is just not possible. Then one thing you can do is to space out how often you get these treatments. On average hair grows about ½ an inch per month, sometimes more, sometimes less. It's much harder to limit the application of relaxer or hair color to a small ½ inch strip of hair than it is to limit it to a 1½ inch strip. Getting frequent touch-ups increases the risk of damaging the hair that has already been treated because it is accidentally being treated twice. Spacing out treatments also gives you more opportunities to strengthen your hair between touch-ups with protein and deep conditioning treatments.

Certainly, all of this may be much easier said than done, but it's yet another simple tweak to your hair care regimen that could pay dividends in the long run.

Twenty-One

Avoid Formaldehyde Containing Keratin Treatments

One of the most common questions I get asked from doctors and patients alike is, "Are keratin treatments safe?" or "Is a keratin treatment safer than a relaxer"? The short answer is: I have no idea. That's because there are so many different formulations and very little is known about the long term side effects of the treatments, so we will start with the fundamentals.

WHAT IS A KERATIN TREATMENT?

Formaldehyde, the main ingredient of the original Brazilian keratin treatment, is a toxin that in high quantities is considered to be a cancer-causing agent. Rumor is, it was discovered as a straightening agent when a Brazilian undertaker noticed that his corpse's hair had straightened on his forearms after he spilled some embalming fluid on the skin. In practice, keratin treatments are a mixture of liquid keratin (similar to the keratin in our hair) and formaldehyde. When the formaldehyde is applied to wet hair, it allows the liquid keratin to link up with the natural keratin and forms a temporary bond while the hair is manually placed in a straight state. To seal the bonds in this straightened formation, intense heat is applied to the hair, and it needs to remain in this position for 48–72 hours. When this heat is applied, formaldehyde gas is released into the hair, and this can be inhaled into the lungs which is concerning.

People like keratin treatments for two reasons:

1) Unlike a relaxer treatment, the straightening results are temporary, lasting 3–4 months at a time. Women are not forced to commit to a straight style, and this lack of long-term commitment can be very tempting.
2) Keratin treatments, unlike relaxer treatments, can be performed the same day as other treatments such as hair coloring. This is because it does not directly impact the inner part of the hair shaft, called the cortex.

The downsides of keratin treatments, though, require some thought. For example, no one knows just how much formaldehyde is being released into the hair during keratin treatments. Because of this, the cancer potential is unknown. All clients receiving this treatment must be okay with this risk

Additionally, over time, keratin treatments damage the hair due to the intense heat required to place the hair in a straightened configuration, especially for those women who are naturally curly.

While there are keratin treatments that market themselves as "formaldehyde-free," these treatments often contain ingredients (such as methylene glycol, glyoxylic acid, and cyclopentasiloxane) that release the same gases during the straightening process. Truly formaldehyde-free keratin treatments do exist but do not provide the same straightening effects as traditional keratin treatments.

Lastly, don't let the term "keratin treatment" fool you. These treatments DO NOT make the hair stronger, and they are not the same as a protein treatment. The term keratin treatment just sounds way more friendly than the alternatives. Because let's be honest, how comfortable would you feel telling your girlfriends that you're on your way to get an "Embalming Fluid Treatment"? Exactly.

Twenty-Two

Avoid Tight Hairstyles

When it comes to hair loss, one of the most vulnerable areas to lose hair is along the temples. It is here that most women notice hair thinning after pregnancy, as they age, and when wearing tight hairstyles. The first two cannot be avoided, but fortunately, the last one can. Tight hairstyles, including tight ponytails, braided extensions, weaves, dreadlocks, and wigs, can all pull out the hair over time. While some women can wear beautifully braided hairstyles again and again with no issue, for most people this will lead to hair loss with repeated use.

One of my favorite phrases is "hair loss begets hair loss." And what I mean by this is the exact styles that we use to cover up hair loss are often the same ones that make hair loss worse. Wigs are notorious for pulling out hair along the hairline, especially when they are glued in place. Over time, dreadlocks can also pull out the hairline, especially when they are freshened up on a regular basis. While this keeps them looking "neat," over time, this can pull out the hair and gradually move your hairline backward.

If you are used to wearing one of these styles and have not experienced hair loss (or you have, and it's just a little bit), then that is great. Early on, hair loss from tightly braided styles is reversible and will grow back with just a little TLC. If you have noticed thinning hair for only a few years, without any shiny bald patches, then it's possible that an over the counter treatment, like minoxidil (see chapter 32) can help. Over time, however, the hair loss can be severe and permanent. At this stage, often the only thing that will grow the hair back is a hair transplant, and those cost anywhere between $10k-$30k. Ask yourself, are your extensions really worth all that? While you are reading this book focusing on improving the strength and length of your hair, do not forget about your hairline. Here are some easy tips you can follow to minimize stress to this sensitive area:

1. Avoid applying extensions to chemically straightened hair. Chemically straightened hair is already weakened, so it makes sense that adding extensions increases the chances of hair loss.
2. Consider extensions that apply less tension to your hairline, like low buns and loose ponytails.
3. Use a satin lined wig cap and draw it forward, slightly past your hairline to minimize breakage.
4. If you wear dreadlocks, extend the time between touch up sessions so that you are re-twisting less often.
5. Before adding weaved extensions, braid cornrows in a horizontal or circular direction around the scalp, instead of vertically, from front to back, to minimize pulling the hair backward away from the hairline.

Twenty-Three

Wear Buns More Often

Without a doubt, my favorite hairstyle for women working their way back to healthy hair is a classic bun. A bun is great for two reasons:

1. It keeps hair from dragging along your shoulders and getting snagged on clothing
2. It protects the ends of your hair which are prone to getting damaged

Additionally, because a bun looks excellent even when "messy," women are less likely to use damaging styling tools to achieve this look. When done correctly, buns should not be tight or held back with multiple clips. This can lead to hair breakage and defeat the purpose of protecting the hair.

If you're looking to grow your hair longer, you will need to emphasize protecting the most vulnerable part of your hair, the ends. If you are looking to grow your hair out, I recommend wearing your hair in a bun about 90 percent of the time and doing a more fun style on the weekends or during special occasions.

An alternative to buns are braided styles that tuck in your ends such as Dutch or halo braids, and high ponytails that don't drag against your clothes. This is one minor style adjustment that has the potential to make a big difference for you in the long run.

Twenty-Four

Beware Weaves, Wigs, and Clip-Ins

Extensions...gotta love them. I love extensions for their ability to virtually eliminate the need for daily hair upkeep. This is especially important to women with curly or kinky hair, which is more prone to damage from routine styling such as combing and brushing. Remember those movies from the 1950s with women insisting that 100 brushstrokes to the hair at night is a recipe for beautiful hair? More like a recipe for disaster, especially if you're a curly-haired girl like me.

Extensions circumvent the need for daily styling and, even better; can transform your hair into the hair of your dreams. Have naturally thin locks but want to look like you have a head full of hair? Extensions can do that. Want blonde hair, but you're a natural brunette? Extensions can do that too. The great part is, you could change your style on nearly a daily basis, so no long-term commitment is necessary!

But this beauty often comes at a price. What may start out as just as a simple preference can eventually become a necessity. That is because all extensions-wigs, weaves, clip-in and braids-can pull out the hair. Hair breakage is more likely if the extensions are attached to hair that has been chemically processed, but can happen anyway.

Clip-in extensions are the easiest to camouflage because only 1 or 2 pieces is needed at a time to increase density. But the tiny comb attachments often rip the hair when they are removed. On top of that, even though clip-ins are designed to be worn for an hour or so at the most, many women keep them in for days (and sometimes months) because they can be very tricky to install. Stylists are typically the ones to install clip-ins, and because it's hard to replicate the work at home, many women are afraid to take them out and end up with clumps of hair on the floor when they are removed.

Wigs are also gaining more popularity, particularly the lace front variety. Lace front wigs are much more natural looking than the wigs your grandmother wore and can be applied very quickly. Most lace fronts are attached with glue or tape, and this tends to wreak havoc on the hairline. Cheap glue is also more likely to lead to hair loss. Over time, the hair loss along the hairline can become permanent, which makes users even more dependent on wigs to cover up the hair loss.

Similar hair loss occurs when sewn-in weaves are applied too often or left in for too long. Ideally weaves should stay in for 2–4 weeks as hair breakage is almost certain to occur if left longer than that. That is because hair, especially curly hair, needs constant moisture to stay healthy. It's nearly impossible to give your hair TLC when it's braided down under a weave for 2–3 months.

Weave fusion styles cause the most damage because, the weave is literally glued to small pieces of your own hair and requires removal by a hair stylist. Sometimes, these fused pieces can fall out on their own and take your hair with it. This form of weave is particularly expensive because it is the most natural appearing extension, but is also the most dangerous.

Still struggling to give up your fave extension hairstyle? Here are my tips on getting the best bang for your buck from extensions:

1. Avoid clip-ins altogether if you can, it's almost impossible to avoid breakage. If you do decide to use clip-ins, limit their use to special events and leave them in place for only a few hours at a time. Leaving them in for days is more likely to lead to tangling and hair damage.
2. Limit the use of weaves to 6 weeks max. Do your absolute best to wash your hair at least every 2–3 weeks while wearing your weave

and apply leave-in conditioner daily if your hair is naturally dry or damaged.

3. Avoid applying extensions such as braids or weaves to hair that has been chemically processed.

4. Try safer alternatives to long term extensions like faux ponytails or faux buns. These can be tied directly onto your own ponytail to give your hair a fuller look and are easy to apply even for the most inexperienced hair styler.

5. Try hair filler fibers if you are trying to camouflage hair thinning, particularly along the front part of your hair. These fibers are designed to attach onto your own hair and give you the appearance of fuller hair.

6. Apply wigs over a satin lined wig cap to protect your hairline. Apply oil to your hairline as well for added protection.

7. If you are using a long term style like weave, give your hair extra TLC for at least 4 weeks (protein treatment, deep condition, etc.) before your next style.

Twenty-Five

Cut Back on Heat Styling

I am going to go out on a limb and guess that, almost every person reading this book owns either a blow-dryer, flat iron or both. These tools continue to be some of the most popular hair styling tools regardless of hair type. Heat styling tools have evolved over the past few decades and now it's easy to find blow dryers and flat irons that *claim* to eliminate all damage and even make your hair healthier (insert skeptical face here).

Well, I will tell you right now, that that is false. But one of the upsides of flat ironing the hair straight is that it allows all of the hair to lie in one direction. This allows light to hit in a way that enhances shine, an effect that is magnified after the use of hair serums, which often contain silicone to add even more shine to the hair. As most of us know, the shine is short lived and gone by the next day and should definitely not be mistaken for a sign of health.

Flat-ironing takes advantage of the hair shaft's ability to temporarily change shape by breaking the hair's hydrogen bonds. Applying water (H_2O) to the hair restores the hydrogen bonds and returns the hair to its natural wavy or curly state. However, healthy hair burns at 451.4 degrees Fahrenheit and damaged hair burns at much lower temperatures. Once the hair burns, the damage is irreversible, and it cannot be restored to health. Even if your hair is not completely burned from one treatment, heat styling does damage the hair and that damage continues to add up each time heat is used. This is because each time the hair is exposed to heat, water is rapidly pushed out of the hair and in the process leaves holes in the hair that leave it fragile and more prone to damage.

So what should you do if you just can't find a way to give up the heat? Try these adjustments:

1. Consider air-drying your hair for as long as possible before blow drying (more on that later): the less water that is pushed out of the hair by a blow dryer, the less damage you will experience. Wait until your hair is at least 75–80 percent dry before reaching for your blow dryer.

2. Try a ceramic or titanium coated flat iron which can lessen damage during flat-ironing by minimizing friction.

3. Cut down the number of times you blow dry and flat iron your hair drastically. If you are experiencing a lot of breakage, then using heat on a regular basis will make things much worse. Consider cutting back on your heat styling by half and eventually decreasing the use to a couple of times a month at the most.

4. Use a heat protectant every time you use heat: These help decrease the amount of heat transferred to the hair during the straightening process.

5. Set your flat iron to 350 degrees or less when straightening your hair.

6. Deep condition your hair before every flat-ironing session because, as always, dry hair is more prone to damage. Flat ironing dry hair is like dropping a match in a dry forest – prepare to watch a burn. Treating your hair to an intense moisturizing session allows it to withstand more heat and thereby minimizes damage.

7. Blow dry your hair on a cool setting: You can do this by pulling the hair taut while blow drying on cool air and still get the hair pretty straight, with much less damage.

8. Like wearing your hair straight every day, but you weren't born with straight hair? Then choose a permanent straightener such as a chemical relaxer or other straightening treatments instead.

These treatments are designed to chemically alter the pattern of your hair so you won't have to straighten your hair artificially on a daily basis. In the end, the damage you experience from these treatments is likely to be less than the damage from blow drying and flat-ironing your hair daily.

If all of this fails and you continue to experience breakage and split ends from using heat, then listen to your hair and drop heat for good. Some people, especially those with thin, fine hair, may just not be able to withstand the damage associated with heat. And you know what they tell you to do if you can't stand the heat...

Twenty-Six

Trim Your Split Ends Regularly

While long hair is not the goal for all women, I do realize that the goal for many women reading this book will be to grow their hair to longer lengths. Long hair comes with its own issues; specifically that it requires more maintenance than short hair. The most common mistake I see women making in their journey to long hair is refusing to cut off frayed, split ends.

It may sound counterintuitive, but if you want long hair, you have to get comfortable with cutting your hair. Split ends are the result of repetitive trauma to the hair. This leads to the loss of the outer portion of the hair, called the cuticle, which exposes the inner portion of the hair, the cortex. While conditioners can temporarily mend split ends, they cannot repair them completely, and over time the split ends can travel up the hair cause the hair to break at higher points along the hair shaft. Things like chemical relaxers, hair color, and heat styling all increase the risk of getting split ends.

When you get regular trims, you can cut off the split ends before they travel up the hair shaft thus minimizing the number of hairs that will be broken off at shorter lengths.

This leads to the inevitable question: how often should one trim the hair? Like almost everything in this book, it depends.

As discussed earlier, hair grows at approximately ½ an inch per month, though this varies from person to person and differs even among people of different ethnic groups. Generally, hair grows a bit faster in people of Asian descent and a little slower in people of African descent. If your hair grows pretty quickly, you may need to trim split ends as often as every 6–8 weeks. If your hair grows more slowly and it is well conditioned and healthy, you may only need to trim every 3–4 months. If the point is to grow your hair, you certainly don't want to trim ½ an inch every 6 weeks, or it would take you years to grow your hair to your shoulders!

How much you trim depends on how much damage you have. If you have not trimmed your hair in a year, you may need to lose a few inches needed to get you back on track. Generally, trimming off about ¼ inch-½ inch per trim should do the trick. A more time consuming but length-conserving method, is to go strand by strand snipping off only split ends, this is called "dusting." In each dusting session, you will only cut off the very ends of the hair. If you prefer this method, you will need to dust often, but you can space out the time between more standard trims. Over time, you may be able to conserve more length this way. Trims can be done at home with hair shears or with a trusted stylist. When done correctly, trimming is the true definition of gaining by losing.

Twenty-Seven

Start Air-Drying Your Hair

Air drying is one of those styling habits that pretty much everyone recognizes as better for their hair, but is rarely done due to the less than stellar results. It's true, blow drying or flat ironing the hair will allow the hair to be straighter than when it's allowed to air dry, especially if you have naturally wavy, curly or tightly curled hair. That being said, there are good reasons to consider making the switch from heat drying to air drying.

We have already discussed the effects that heat has on the hair. As you recall, healthy hair burns at 451.4°F (233°C), but damage occurs at much lower levels than this. Like flat ironing, blow drying the hair can lead to damage that builds up over time. If you are looking for fuller hair adding air drying to your hair regimen can drastically improve the strength of your hair.

There are many ways to air dry your hair so that the end result is similar to blow drying. These differ based on your natural hair type. If you are looking for different techniques to try, I suggest you browse YouTube, a treasure trove of hair tips and techniques.

Committing to air drying 100 percent is perhaps one of the most challenging tips in this book, mostly because it's difficult to completely replicate a look achieved with blow dryers and flat irons.

If you don't think you're quite ready to make the switch, there are at least two ways to incorporate air drying into your routine without eliminating heat styling cold turkey:

1. Consider alternating days you blow dry your hair with days you air dry. This essentially cuts down your use of heat styling tools in half. Consider limiting blow drying to days when you have events or special occasions.
2. Air dry your hair until it is 75–85 percent dry and then blow dry the rest on a warm or cool setting.

If you can commit to air drying even a little bit, your hair will thank you with more shine and density in the long run.

Twenty-Eight

Try Nightly Scalp Massages for Hair Growth

There are a few treatments that I mention in this book that have not been researched extensively by the scientific community and scalp massage is one of them. However, the risks are so low and with the potential for benefits existing, it falls into my "Can't Hurt" category.

Here's the theory behind scalp massages: scalp massages are thought to increase blood flow in the scalp, and that increased blood flow could, in theory, help stimulate hair growth. A quick search of scalp massagers will yield dozens of results of awkward looking contraptions that promise to stimulate hair growth. However, if you are interested in trying scalp massage, I recommend using the original scalp massager: your fingers. A few minutes a day should suffice, and if there is improvement, you should notice it within a couple of months. Some people enjoy adding oils to the scalp prior to the scalp massage, including essential oils like peppermint and tea tree oil (diluted, of course), both of which lead to some refreshing tingling of the scalp as well.

Best case scenario, you notice some hair growth and worst case scenario, it doesn't work. Either way, scalp massages are great stress relievers so you should at least feel more relaxed, and who doesn't love that?

Twenty-Nine

Try Steaming Your Hair

With all of this talk about how terrible heat is for your strands, you would assume that hair steamers would be a terrible idea, but that's not true. While dry heat in the form of flat irons and blow dryers can dry out your hair and lead to breakage, moist heat can actually be great for your hair. Moist heat encourages the scales on your hair's cuticles to lift up and welcome more moisture which leads to more resilience and less breakage.

Steaming treatments are ideal for hair that is very dry or damaged. If you are chemically styling your hair by using relaxers, bleach or dye, then a regular steaming treatment may go a long way. There are a few steamers that can be purchased online, but steaming treatments are also commonly done in salons.

To incorporate steaming into your regimen, apply your deep conditioner as you normally would during your hair washing session. Instead of letting your deep conditioner sit under a shower cap alone, sit under a steamer (with or without a shower cap) to allow the moist heat to open up your cuticles and moisturize your strands. You can also steam your hair without a deep conditioner and just allow the moist water to moisturize your hair.

It's important not to overuse a hair steamer. Too much of anything is bad after a while. Some people may notice that if their hair is over moisturized it feels limp and lifeless and will not hold onto styles well. Figure out your ideal steaming frequency by playing around with your regimen. To begin with, I would recommend trying steaming treatments monthly then increasing frequency as needed.

Thirty

Sleep with a Satin
Pillowcase at Night
to Curb Hair Breakage

E ver woken up to broken hairs on your pillowcase? I know I have. By
this point in the book, you have seen me go on and on about the
importance of keeping your hair well hydrated and moisturized. Well most
pillowcases, especially those made of cotton, help achieve just the opposite. This is because cotton does a great job of wicking moisture away
from surfaces and tends to be pretty rough compared to satin and silk.
Ever been splashed in a cotton shirt? It dries pretty quickly. Get splashed
in a satin shirt, and you'll feel soaked for hours. Cotton also tends to be
rough and the constant friction from tossing and turning can be enough
to break fragile hair strands. Switching to a satin or silk pillowcase will
minimize the breakage you experience overnight. Similarly, wearing a silk
or satin headscarf or cap at night will have the same effect and also help
preserve hairstyles overnight.

While this may seem like a minor adjustment, sleeping with a satin
cap or pillowcase can be a game-changer for those with curly hair for
whom keeping the hair moisturized is of utmost importance. You can easily find satin lined saps at beauty supply stores and satin pillowcases for
purchase online.

Thirty-One

Use a Heat Protectant

In this book, I devote multiple chapters to heat styling because it is one of the most common ways in which we damage our hair on a regular basis. Heat damage can come in the form of blow dryers, flat irons and styles like Brazilian keratin treatments. Typically, to straighten the hair, heating tools are set anywhere between 300 and 500 degrees to achieve the desired result. At the higher end of this temperature range, it is not unusual to visualize steam leaving the hair while it is being straightened. Not only does this weaken the hair, but it can actually irreversibly damage the hair. One method of minimizing the damage your hair experiences during the straightening process,0 is to use a heat protectant before you flat iron or blow dry your hair.

Heat protectants are typically made of silicones or other chemicals that coat the hair and decrease the amount of heat that is directly transferred to the hair shaft. This then minimizes the extent of damage the hair experiences during each styling session.

However, even with a heat protectant, I recommend limiting the temperature on your flat iron to a maximum of 350 degrees when using it.

If you find that you are having too tough of a time cutting back on your heat styling, incorporate this tip into your regimen and see if helps decrease breakage over time. If not, you may have no choice but to bid your favorite flat iron adieu.

Thirty-Two

Try Minoxidil for
Thinning Hair

Minoxidil is the only FDA approved treatment for a type of hormonal hair loss called androgenetic alopecia, also known as male or female pattern balding. In women, this usually leads to progressive hair loss on the temples, in the front or central portion of the scalp. While it is not recommended on areas of frank hair loss, where the scalp feels smooth, minoxidil can be helpful in areas of thinning.

To understand how minoxidil works, you have to understand a little bit about hair biology. A typical hair follicle has three phases: a growing phase (called the anagen phase), a resting phase (catagen) and a shedding phase (telogen). In hair that has been affected by hormonal thinning, the growing phase is much shorter, and the hair grows in much thinner than usual. Over time, a collection of thin hairs makes it look like there is less hair present, thus making the scalp more visible. Minoxidil returns hair back to its normal growth characteristics, meaning it will grow back thicker and stay in the growing phase for more extended periods of time.

Sounds great right? It can be, for the right person. Here are some potential downsides you should consider before rushing off to buy a bottle of minoxidil:

1. Minoxidil only works for certain types of hair loss. Pattern balding is the classic hair loss it works for, but it can also work for

people who have lost the hair along their temples from wearing tight extensions. Before trying minoxidil, you should ask your dermatologist if you have the type of hair loss that would respond to minoxidil. If you don't, you may just end up wasting money and feel disappointed with your results.

2. While using minoxidil, you may notice that your hair loss looks worse before it looks better. That is because minoxidil pushes out all of the hair that is not growing correctly. If you are not comfortable with this prospect, then minoxidil may not be for you.

3. Minoxidil only works while you are using it. Think of your hair like a plant and minoxidil as water. If you water a plant every day for two years, it will look lush and grow. But if you suddenly stop watering that plant for a month, it will wither away as if you never nourished it for two years prior. Minoxidil works in the same way. While you will not need to use it every day forever, stopping cold turkey for a month or longer will lead to loss of results.

4. Even with the right type of hair loss, minoxidil may not work. I still consider it the most reliable medical treatment for hair thinning, but it only leads to hair growth in about half of its users. If you notice no improvement after three months, then it's best to stop using it.

Minoxidil is not a cure for hair loss, but it can work well if you are willing to be patient.

Thirty-Three

Try an Essential Oil Blend
for Hair Growth

A s I have mentioned before, very few oils have been studied by the medical community for their benefits on the hair. One of the few exceptions is an essential oil blend which was studied for a form of hair loss called alopecia areata. In alopecia areata, the body's cells, designed to attack bacteria and viruses, begin to attack the hair follicle instead, leading to coin-shaped patches on the scalp. In a study published in the Archives of Dermatology (now called JAMA Dermatology) half of the patients with alopecia areata were treated with the essential oil blend and the other half were treated with a placebo consisting just of grape seed and jojoba oil. After seven months they noticed more patients treated with the essential oil blend (44%) had at least some hair growth compared to those who used the placebo blend (6%).

Before you decide if you would like to try this mixture yourself, remember that even though essential oils are available over the counter, they can still cause severe allergic reactions, especially if not diluted with inactive/carrier oils first. Before you start, apply the combination oil behind your ear to see if you react. If you notice a reaction, then this may not be for you.

Also, in general, essential oils should be avoided by women who are pregnant, have high blood pressure, a history of seizures or other chronic medical conditions. Get approval from your doctor first before trying any new treatment.

Essential Oil Blend For Hair Growth
2 drops thyme oil
3 drops lavender oil
3 drops rosemary oil
2 drops cedarwood oil
3 mL jojoba oil
20 mL grape seed oil

Combine all oils as listed above into one container. Massage three drops into thinning areas for two minutes. Cover with a warm towel afterward for 10–15 minutes. Repeat every night.

As with all things regarding hair, this method requires patience; ingredients can be tough to find, and it may take months to see hair growth. All that aside, if you are a fan of essential oils this may be worth a try.

Thirty-Four

Give Castor Oil a Try for Hair Growth

There is perhaps no other oil that has as much hype attached to it as castor oil. Castor oil, made from pressed castor beans, has been used for centuries for hair growth, though the actual benefits of castor oil are unknown. In fact, while there are dozens of patent applications for the use of castor oil for the hair, there are no scientific studies that have assessed whether or not castor oil actually promotes hair growth. However, I put castor oil firmly into the "Can't Hurt" category. Castor oil can be purchased for just a few dollars at any organic health store or beauty supply store. It is a very thick and viscous oil so if you have fine hair that is easily weighed down by products, this product is likely not for you. To use castor oil, rub a small amount to thinning areas twice a day. If you see no results within three months, then you should stop use.

Even if you do not notice hair growth, that does not mean you should throw your castor oil in the trash. Castor oil has great moisturizing qualities and can be added to deep conditioners to boost moisturizing potential and can also be applied to wet hair after washing to keep the hair feeling moisturized longer.

Thirty-Five

Apply Coconut Oil to Your Hair Before and After Washing

C oconut oil should be a staple on the beauty shelf for anyone reading this book and has more scientific data supporting its use for the hair than probably any other oil. Coconut oil is most helpful when used as a part of your hair wash routine because it has a unique chemical structure that allows it to penetrate deeply into the hair shaft. As a result, coconut oil has the ability to minimize the swelling and breakage that occurs when washing the hair, a phenomenon termed *hygral fatigue.*

Coconut oil can also help with your post-wash routine. As I mentioned before, washing the hair can lead to breakage and weaken the hair shaft. But coconut oil has actually been shown to minimize post-wash hair protein loss and improve moisture retention, thus leading to stronger hair.

I should mention that there are some people who feel that their hair does not react well when coconut oil is applied to it, and if that is the case for you, that is okay. Unfortunately, while many oils may help with moisture retention, most have a molecular size that is too large to penetrate the hair shaft in the same way that coconut oil does.

I recommend using coconut oil as below:

1. Apply softened coconut oil to dry hair and cover with a shower cap or warm towel for 10–15 minutes.

2. Shampoo and condition the hair as normal.
3. Apply coconut oil immediately after washing. Alternatively, you can apply a water-based (for straight, wavy or thin hair) or cream based (thick, curly hair) leave-in conditioner to the hair if your hair is dry before applying coconut oil.

One last note: there are many different types of coconut oil available: virgin, refined, processed, unprocessed and a combination of these four. I generally recommend organic, virgin coconut oil whether it has been processed or not. You can play around with different varieties and figure out what works best for you.

Thirty-Six

Add Apple Cider Vinegar to Your Shampoo

Ever wonder why getting your hair washed in a salon turns out much better than when you do it at home? It's partially because salon grade shampoos are made to be slightly acidic, with a pH of 5, while most shampoos we use at home have neutral to slightly basic charge >7. It may not seem like such a huge deal, but it can have a significant impact on your hair.

If you recall from chemistry (more science, I know), acids are positively charged while basic solutions are negatively charged. A positive charge on the hair actually minimizes frizz and increases shine and luster. Ever had hat hair? That's what happens when your hair is loaded with negative charges; it's a fly-away bonanza.

Using shampoo alone leaves negative charges on the hair and conditioners, which are positively charged, balance that out and effectively neutralize the charge on your hair.

It's tough (and expensive) to get access to salon grade shampoos, but one easy fix is to add apple cider vinegar to your shampoo. Shampooing your hair with a slightly acidic shampoo can increase the shine and luster in your hair. Vinegar is naturally acidic and when mixed with shampoo can create a gentle acid based shampoo that minimizes frizz and flyaways. I recommend starting with a ¼ cup of ACV in a full bottle of shampoo. You can also use apple cider vinegar alone to cleanse your hair, but it must be diluted with water first. Applying plain apple cider vinegar directly to the hair is too acidic and may irritate your skin.

Thirty-Seven

Try an Ayurvedic Treatment

Natural remedies are loved by almost everyone. I love them too, and I occasionally incorporate essential oils and ayurvedic treatments into my daily regimen. There are two important things to remember about natural treatments, and I would be remiss if I didn't mention them here:

1) Herbal remedies do not go through the rigorous testing that prescription medications do to ensure that they are safe or effective. In that sense, taking them is much riskier than taking or using a prescription medication.
2) Just because something is natural does not mean it's safe. Cocaine is completely natural and far from being safe.

Now that we have that out of the way, I believe there is a role for many natural hair treatments in routine hair care, a few of which I discuss below. As a medical doctor, I am obviously a strong proponent of modern medicine. However, the fact is that when it comes to hair, there is still so much we have to learn. I am asked all the time about natural remedies and whether they are effective, especially whether they will make the hair grow.

AYURVEDIC TREATMENTS FOR HEALTHY HAIR

Shikakai powder: Shikakai is a plant that is native to Southern India and has been used for generations as a natural cleansing agent. In Hindi, it translates to "fruit of the hair" and contains natural saponins which allow it to lather like regular shampoo. However, unlike regular shampoo, it actually leaves the hair feeling more conditioned after use. It is naturally acidic and, as I discussed previously, this leaves the hair with increased shine and decreased flyaways. One downside is that it is very grainy and to remove all the grains you will likely need to spend a much longer time actually washing your hair. You may even continue to notice very fine in your grains a few days later. However, if you are willing to withstand this small annoyance, shikakai is more than worth the trouble.

Amla: Amla, also known as Indian gooseberry, is a popular ingredient in hair care products around the world. Also originating in the Indian subcontinent, you can now find amla in the form of oils and shampoos as it is a great natural moisturizer.

Reetha: Reetha is a natural soapnut that is native to south Asia and is often combined with amla and shikakai to form a natural, moisturizing shampoo. While historically these shampoos were made by immersing the three in water for several hours, you can purchase ready-made versions of shampoos containing these ingredients online.

Thirty-Eight

Replace Your Hair Dye with Henna

Henna, also known as Lawsone, is considered one of the original hair dyes and has been around for over 3,000 years. The most common form of henna is used to dye the hair reddish-orange and is commonly used to cover gray hairs. Like most natural hair dyes, the response is subtle and requires multiple treatments over time to achieve desired results.

One major downside of henna application is that it is tedious and messy. Henna stains the skin and hair very easily and is commonly used to create beautiful, elaborate hand tattoos that can take weeks to wash away. It is this staining property that makes it both an effective dye and a hassle to apply.

Henna typically comes as a greenish powder which is then mixed with an acid (orange juice, apple cider vinegar, etc.) into a thick paste and then left to sit for several minutes to hours to release the dye. This paste is then applied to the hair and should be allowed to sit for at least 30 minutes to help transfer color to the hair. True natural henna can make the hair feel dry and brittle afterward and so following with a deep conditioner is recommended.

Because henna is actually just "staining" the hair, there is very little damage associated with this dye treatment, and for this reason, it is a healthier alternative to coloring the hair. That being said, natural henna will only create a reddish-orange color that may not be desirable to many people. Now, many companies have started marketing henna coloring kits that create a variety of shades (such as black henna), and most of these contain chemicals found in other hair dyes. This includes the ingredient para-phenylenediamine (PPD) which can cause allergic reactions. Some brands that are marketed as natural henna still have this ingredient, so you should always test your skin for sensitivity before applying henna to the entire scalp. Indigo powder is another form of natural hair dye that can be used to dye the hair a bluish-black color but also can be mixed with henna to form a brownish color.

A different form of henna, Cassia obovota, is commonly known as a henna gloss treatment. This treatment does not dye the hair but has some conditioning properties that may decrease hair breakage. Like regular henna, the benefits build up over time and typically a gloss treatment is applied every 4–6 weeks for maximum benefit.

Thirty-Nine

Try Using Lemon Juice to Lighten Your Hair

As we have discussed, it is challenging to lighten the hair without experiencing damage, as most temporary dyes can only make the hair darker. One natural alternative is to try lemon juice to lighten the hair. While it will not turn you from a brunette to a blonde, lemon juice can lighten your hair a couple of shades, especially if you are willing to be patient and try it a couple of times.

To do this, you need:

- Lemons (the number varies based on how much hair you have)
- Water
- Lots of sunlight

Mix equal amounts of lemon juice and water and place it in a spray bottle. Spray the lemon juice mixture over the entire area you are trying to lighten. After spraying your hair, you will need at least a couple of hours of direct sunlight. Plan to try this treatment on a day when you expect to be outdoors, whether that is watching a baseball game or running a marathon.

A word of caution: this treatment can be very drying, so I do not recommend this if you are dealing with a lot of damage. Also, you should plan for a deep conditioning treatment once you have spent the requisite amount of time outdoors. Alternatively, you can mix your favorite conditioner in your lemon juice/water mixture to minimize the drying effects.

For most people, multiple treatments will be required before you start to notice a difference. However, if you notice dryness and breakage after your first treatment, it's best to avoid repeating it in the future.

Forty

Dye Your Hair Brown with Coffee

Looking for another fun way to dye your hair? Consider using coffee to turn your hair darker. This technique basically takes advantage of coffee's ability to stain the hair.

To try this, you will need the following:

- Instant coffee mix
- Conditioner
- Applicator brush (you can get this from a beauty supply store)

Mix equal amounts of instant coffee mix and conditioner in a bowl. You want the final mixture to look dark, so if you need to, you can use extra instant coffee mix. Use the applicator brush to brush on thick layers of the coffee/conditioner mixture onto your hair. Leave in place for one to two hours before rinsing out.

Like other natural hair dye options, the results may be subtle at first, and it may take a few tries before you notice improvement. All that being said, if you are just looking for darker hair color with minimal damage, then temporary hair rinses are still a better option. But if you are looking for a chemical-free alternative, the coffee is an excellent option for you.

Forty-One

Repurpose Breakfast Food into a Protein-Packed Hair Treatment

I f you are someone who prefers to make their own products at home from scratch, then you will be happy to learn that some of your favorite foods can be applied to the hair to help strengthen them and add shine to your hair.

Here are some of my favorite breakfast foods that double as hair products:

1. Eggs: Most people are familiar with eggs as a protein-based addition to their diet. Similarly, eggs can be used as a hair mask to help strengthen your hair. While most of the protein in eggs is likely too big to penetrate the hair shaft, many users of egg masks do report hair that feels stronger with regular use.

   To use, make sure you beat the eggs well before applying to the hair. Like other protein treatments, the egg mixture should be left on the hair for 10–15 minutes, preferably with a source of heat. Consider adding conditioner or other moisturizing products to the egg mixture to avoid having it dry out your hair too much. Of course, you have to take extra care to make sure that you do not eat any raw egg product as this could lead to infection with

Salmonella, a dangerous bacteria that is a common cause of food poisoning.

2. Avocado: Avocados are packed with natural fats and oils that make them a great moisturizer for the hair. They also have a moderate amount of amino acids (protein) that allow it to serve as a dual moisturizing and strengthening treatment. The hair benefits of avocado have been recognized for quite some time, and for this reason, avocado oil is a popular oil, that you can purchase on its own, to help hold in moisture and add shine to the hair.

    To use, mash up one avocado (or two, depending on your hair length and density) and apply it directly to your hair. Leave on for 15–30 minutes. Consider adding it to your favorite conditioner for a more luxurious deep conditioning experience.

3. Bananas: While bananas do not pack as much protein as eggs or avocado, they can serve as an excellent option for light protein treatments. While I would not recommend using them alone, mixing them with other moisturizing ingredients such as honey or olive oil can make for the perfect treatment with a nice balance of protein and moisturizing to ensure your hair feels healthy and not too brittle.

    To use, mash 1–3 bananas with ½ a cup of oil and leave on the hair for 15–30 minutes before rinsing out.

Forty-Two

Add Honey to Your Conditioner for Added Softness

L et's be honest, honey is pretty much good on everything. Turns out, it's also great for your hair. Honey is a rich moisturizer due to its humectant properties. A humectant pulls moisture inward by binding to water in the environment as well as in the hair. Adding honey to your conditioner helps your hair do a better job of absorbing the water and holding onto it for days at a time. Glycerin is another example of a common humectant.

Honey is a great option for women with really dry hair. If you have no problems keeping your hair feeling moisturized or you notice that your hair feels greasy quickly, then you may not like how your hair feels after you add honey.

If you think you may be ready to try honey, start by adding one teaspoon of honey to a cupful of conditioner, and remember, a little goes a long way. I would not recommend applying honey directly to your hair without combining it with a product, or you may just end up with sticky tresses, not to mention you may attract unwelcome guests in the forms of bugs and insects. Proceed wisely!

Forty-Three

Incorporate Caffeine into Your Regimen for Hair Growth

C affeine is one of the few food products that has been studied for its benefits in hair health. Studies have shown that when small hair follicles are removed from the scalp and studied in a petri dish (also known as in vitro) applying caffeine to the hair leads to faster hair growth and a longer growing phase. It may also counteract the progression of female pattern balding though it is unclear how long those benefits would last. Lastly, caffeine can increase blood flow to the scalp and may stimulate hair growth that way.

Many bloggers exalt the benefits of caffeine at reducing hair shedding, especially in periods when hair shedding is expected, such as after giving birth.

You can incorporate caffeine into your hair regimen in many ways, including using it to dye your hair (see Chapter 40), as a midweek spray, and as a rinse. If you are interested in trying a tea rinse, you will need the following:

- Three tea bags (black tea or green tea depending on your preference)
- Water
- Spray bottle

To make your tea rinse, steep three tea bags in a cup of boiling water. Drain the resulting tea into a cup and allow it to cool before transferring to a spray bottle. After shampooing, spray the mixture all over the hair and allow it to sit for at least 5 minutes before moving onto your conditioner or deep conditioner. Repeat with every wash, unless you notice dryness. If that is the case, cut it down to as often as needed until the dryness improves.

Forty-Four

Skip the Biotin

Without a doubt, there is no vitamin supplement that I am asked about more than biotin. Many of my patients reach for biotin as their first go-to when they are experiencing issues with their hair. In fact, many "hair, skin, and nails" vitamins contain biotin as the main ingredient.

THE SCIENCE BEHIND BIOTIN

Biotin is a water-soluble B vitamin that sustains a variety of bodily functions. Babies who are born with a genetic defect that leads to biotin deficiency develop a bright red rash early in life and tend to have sparse hair. Giving these babies biotin can lead to a complete reversal of the rash and improvement in the appearance of their hair. There are other genetic syndromes that lead to hair defects as well, and these are often detectable in infancy. There are studies looking at small groups of patients (sometimes just a handful at a time) that have shown that these kids born with genetic defects notice an improvement in their hair when they take biotin as well. These two things are what have led the cosmetic industry to market biotin to the masses as the holy grail for hair loss. Some studies have also shown an improvement in nail strength in healthy adults taking biotin supplements.

One big problem: No studies have shown the benefit of biotin in improving hair quality in healthy adults without genetic defects.

This is a big reason why many people get frustrated with biotin, especially if they are having trouble growing their hair or they are experiencing a lot of breakage. It does very little, if anything at all, at improving the hair. At least not in the way that people hope it to work. I tell my patients that at best, their hair may get a little stronger but it certainly won't grow faster or shine more.

THE DANGERS OF BIOTIN

The really concerning thing about biotin is that when taken in high levels it can actually interfere with many lab studies. For example, taking a biotin supplement can falsely impact your thyroid studies leading some to believe that you have an overactive thyroid gland. While there are other studies that can confirm or deny this, for a brief time you may think you have thyroid disease.

What's more worrisome is that taking excess biotin can actually mask the lab test that doctors rely on to diagnose a heart attack. When you have a heart attack, your body releases select chemicals into your bloodstream, including one called troponin. High levels of troponin are critical to diagnosing a heart attack, but biotin interferes with troponin testing and falsely lowers troponin levels even if they are actually high. Recently, the FDA put out a bulletin warning patients about taking biotin after a patient died because their heart attack could not be properly diagnosed for this reason. While the specifics of the case are unclear, you should know that chest pain is not enough to diagnose a heart attack, and its symptoms can be similar to a panic attack or even indigestion. Some people experiencing a heart attack may not have chest pain at all and instead, just have numbness in their left arm. Imagine you're at the emergency room with chest pain, sweating bullets, and all your lab tests come back normal because you're taking biotin. You could be sent home when you actually need emergency surgery.

All of this is to say, think twice about taking biotin supplements. The upside is limited, and the downside could be the difference between life and death.

Forty-Five

Take Iron Supplements If You're Deficient

Iron-deficiency anemia is the most common blood disorder among women. Women naturally have lower blood counts, and iron levels than men do, mostly due to monthly menstruation. However, normal iron levels are incredibly important to ensuring healthy hair growth. Many studies have demonstrated the critical importance of iron in regulating healthy hair growth.

Furthermore, low iron levels can lead to rapid hair shedding, a medical condition called telogen effluvium. Telogen effluvium happens at least once to most women in their lifetime, especially within a few months of giving birth, when starting a new medication or at the end of a particularly stressful period in their lives. Fortunately, it's temporary and reverses itself within a couple months of starting.

The exception is in patients with iron deficiency. Low iron levels can cause hair shedding to persist for several months which can be devastating to women. The tough part is, you can be iron deficient and not even know about it. That is because most people with mild iron deficiency will have no symptoms at all, even if it is causing hair loss. Women with severe deficiency will notice that they are excessively tired or are craving things like ice cubes all day.

Here are things you should do if you believe your iron levels are low and may be causing issues with your hair:

1) See your doctor. They can order blood work and can tell you how much iron you need to take to normalize your levels again.
2) Stock up on iron packed foods. These include things like meats (beef, chicken, pork), shellfish (oysters, clams, and mussels in particular), spinach ,or tofu.
3) Drink more orange juice. The vitamin C in orange juice helps you to absorb the iron in your foods better.

If you are low in iron and are working to fix your levels, be patient. It can take months before you notice a difference in your blood work and hair. However, if low iron levels are your problem, you should notice a significant improvement in your hair once your levels improve.

Forty-Six

Check Your Vitamin D Levels

Vitamin D is one of the most important vitamins when it comes to hair health. This vitamin continues to mystify doctors, and we are still learning about all of the benefits of having normal vitamin D levels. Most of the vitamin D in our body comes from exposure to the sun, and some scientists believe that vitamin D is the reason why there are variations in skin tones across the world. For example, it's possible that as humans left Africa, their skin became lighter so they could process as much vitamin D as possible from the little sun they received in northern climates. This potential evolutionary development may hint at the importance of vitamin D.

However, today we know that excess sun exposure can lead to all types of harmful effects: skin cancer, skin discoloration, and wrinkles, to name a few. For these reasons and many others, we spend less time outdoors, and vitamin D deficiency has become common. Fortunately, we can get vitamin D from our diet and through supplements.

While it's unclear if low vitamin D levels are solely responsible for hair loss, there is evidence that it can make whatever hair loss you have worse. Low vitamin D levels have been linked to prolonged shedding that occurs after stressful events and may even worsen hormonal hair loss. Fortunately, vitamin D levels are usually checked annually as part of the routine blood work during checkups with your doctor. If you are unsure of the last time you had your vitamin D levels checked, talk to your physician.

Most low levels of Vitamin D can be brought back to normal with just a daily supplement. Severely low vitamin D levels may require higher doses which are only available through your doctor.

Forty-Seven

Avoid Crash Diets

We've all been there before: we're one month away from a big event: a wedding, prom, or college reunion. We realize we're 10 pounds heavier than we would like to be, so the idea of a crash diet inevitably floats through our minds. There are all types of wacky diets targeted toward women, many of which cause weight loss by drastically altering your body's calorie intake.

One of the early manifestations of prolonged starvation or eating disorders, such as anorexia or bulimia, is hair thinning. The hair is uniquely sensitive to fat loss and nutritional deficiencies. We also know that the base of each hair follicle is surrounded by healthy fat, so fat is essential to healthy hair growth.

Crash diets like juice cleanses (anyone remember Beyoncé's infamous lemon juice and cayenne pepper diet??) are typically used for women who seek quick, short term weight loss. These work by putting the body in a state of prolonged starvation to help burn fat. These diets typically restrict calorie intake to as little as 500 calories a day. The average woman needs at least 3–4 times that amount to sustain basic daily functions underscoring why these types of diets can be both successful and dangerous.

One diet that is gaining in popularity is called the HCG diet. Human chorionic gonadotropin, or HCG for short, is a hormone that is produced early on in pregnancy and helps sustain a healthy pregnancy. It's also the hormone that home pregnancy kits detect when a woman first becomes pregnant. During the HCG diet, clients are instructed to inject HCG into themselves on a daily basis for about two weeks and additionally restrict their calorie intake to 500 calories. After stopping the treatment users don't just notice a thinner waistline, but often a thinner head of hair as well. The rapid shift in hormones (similar to what women experience after pregnancy) plus the dramatic weight loss are a potent combination that stun the hair follicles and send them into a shedding phase. HCG hormone shots are not regulated by the FDA, and the impact on the health is a complete mystery, so, buyers beware.

Now, you would like to think that if women noticed hair loss immediately after a "cleanse" that it would stop them from doing them. The problem is, the hair loss that occurs from rapid nutritional shifts don't manifest as hair loss until 3–6 months later. By that time, many women have difficulty pinpointing the cause.

While losing weight is a difficult task, add hair health to the list of many reasons why losing weight in a slow, steady way, with a healthy diet and plenty of exercise, is the way to go.

Forty-Eight

Pursue Wellness Activities

S tress causes hair loss. I repeat… stress causes hair loss. The type of hair loss often associated with stress is called telogen effluvium. Telogen effluvium is a reversible type of hair loss that occurs during periods of intense physical or mental distress. This stress, especially when experienced in short, high bursts, can be devastating to the hair. Examples of distress include having a baby, major surgery, a death in the family, loss (or start) of a job, ending a romantic relationship and the list goes on. Hair shedding from telogen effluvium can be intense, and it's not unusual for women to report losing handfuls of hair each time they wash, for weeks at a time. So, what may start as an unavoidable life event can be made worse by the hair loss that follows. For this reason, it is important to do whatever it takes to minimize stressors in your life.

This includes exercising, spending time with friends and engaging in any other activities you enjoy. If you are experiencing hair shedding and have eliminated other medical conditions as a potential cause for your hair loss, as crazy as it sounds, try to ignore the hair shedding as much as possible. Counting hair only makes things worse, and some level of shedding on a daily basis is expected. While hair loss may persist for months, it is temporary and will eventually stop. Our hair truly is a reflection of us, and the first step to achieving healthy hair is becoming a healthy you.

Forty-Nine

Get Screened for Conditions That Can Cause Hair Loss

It should go without saying that sometimes hair loss is your body's way of telling you that something is not right. If you have suddenly noticed that you are losing large clumps of hair every time you shower or brush your hair, this could be a sign of something being wrong. Many of the internal causes of hair loss are easily treatable and fortunately reversible, so you should not be afraid of talking to your doctor about your issues.

Below are some common conditions found in women that can manifest as hair loss:

1) Lupus: this is an autoimmune condition in which the parts of your body designed to attack bacteria and viruses (your white blood cells) instead mistakenly begin to attack certain parts of your body. Patients with lupus will often complain of sudden sensitivity to the sunlight, joint pains and feeling excessively tired. Occasionally, they will also notice sudden hair loss that can leave bald patches. While lupus cannot be detected by routine blood work, your doctor can order more specialized blood work that can determine if you have lupus.

2) Thyroid disease: Your thyroid gland plays a vital role in regulating your body's temperature, weight, and energy levels. Patients with thyroid disease may notice sudden hot flashes (not associated

with menopause), rapid weight gain or loss, loss of energy or feeling jittery. Any type of thyroid disease can lead to hair loss, which manifests as increased hair shedding. Women suffering from thyroid disease may notice a slow thinning all over the scalp or may notice large clumps while washing their hair. Thyroid disease is less likely to leave bald patches in the scalp. Since thyroid disease is so common among women, thyroid function is often checked during annual check-ups.

3) Polycystic Ovarian Syndrome (PCOS): PCOS is a complex disease that can be associated with infertility, severe acne and hair loss. Women suffering from PCOS often have irregular periods, and the condition can cause weight gain. While women with PCOS will not necessarily notice hair shedding, they may notice their hair thinning over time, especially at the front and top of the scalp. That is because early presentations of hormonal hair loss or pattern balding, is a common symptom of PCOS. PCOS is more difficult to diagnose because there is not a single blood test that confirms the diagnosis but rather, having a specific set of symptoms in association with certain blood findings (included high testosterone levels) help your doctor make the diagnosis. If you are concerned you may have PCOS, you can talk to your gynecologist about your symptoms and possible treatment options.

While these three conditions are some of the more common conditions that can lead to hair loss, many other conditions may cause hair loss as well. It is important to make sure you are up to date on all of your health screenings as this is critically important not just to your hair health, but your health in general as well.

Fifty

See a Dermatologist

You've reached the end of the book, congratulations! It is my hope that in reading this book you have learned a great deal about what it takes to improve the health of your hair. For a few of you, however, this is less of a happy ending. If you have tried many of the tips found in this book, given it the requisite 90 days, and you still notice issues with your hair, then I strongly recommend you see your dermatologist.

Dermatologists are specially trained at treating diseases of the skin, hair, and nails. There are at least a dozen different types of medical hair loss, and very few can be reversed by what you have read in this book. While this book focuses on caring for the hair after it has left your scalp, a dermatologist can help you determine if you have a medical condition that is hindering hair growth or leading to baldness. You should definitely see a dermatologist if you are experiencing scalp symptoms such as pain, burning or itching in the scalp that doesn't seem to go away no matter what you try. The answer you are searching for may only be a doctor's visit away.

Appendix A

Sample Regimen for Straight/Wavy Damaged Hair

- Wash hair every other day. Either alternate sulfate free shampoo with sulfate containing shampoo or wash with sulfate free shampoo 75 percent of the time.
- Use moisturizing conditioner with every wash.
- Deep Condition the hair with heat at least monthly.
- Once a week, apply a light protein treatment to the hair either before or after shampooing. Cover with a cap for at least 30 minutes before rinsing.

Other considerations:

- Apply a light protein treatment to the hair weekly for a month, then every month for three months. Consider adding at least one salon strength protein treatment every 3 months.
- Alter or eliminate at least one damaging practice
  - o Eliminate flat iron and blow dry on medium heat only
  - o Eliminate permanent color and switch to demi or semi-permanent only

Appendix B

Sample Regimen for Curly/Coily Damaged Hair

- Apply protein treatment to dry or damp hair. Cover with shower cap or heating source for 30 minutes.
- Wash hair once weekly with sulfate free shampoo.
- Deep condition with every shampoo. Follow deep conditioning with moisturizing rinse-out conditioner.
- Add leave in conditioner after washing, at least 3x/week.
- End washing session with light oil.

Other considerations

- Use sulfate containing shampoo a maximum of once monthly.
- For severe damage, you can consider using stronger, salon based protein treatments once monthly.
- Eliminate at least one damaging practice-
  - o Air dry hair whenever possible and limit blow drying and flat ironing to special events only.
  - o Eliminate permanent color and switch to temporary rinses only until damage is eliminated.
  - o Eliminate use of no-lye relaxers. Switch to texturizer or mild relaxers performed in salons only. Stretch relaxers to once every 3 months.

Appendix C

Product Recommendations

These product recommendations are based on personal experience and feedback from my patients. I do not have any financial relationships or endorse any of the listed brands. Remember, it may take a few tries before you find the product of your choice.

Shampoo: Ingredients to look for include cocamidopropyl betaine, decyl glucoside, stearamidopropyl dimethylamine. ***Avoid frequent use of shampoos with sulfates like sodium/ammonium lauryl sulfate, sodium/ammonium laureth sulfate, etc.***

Carol's Daughter Marula Curl Therapy Gentle Cream Cleanser (low-foaming)
Creme of Nature Moisture and Shine Shampoo with Argan Oil
Devacurl Low Poo or No Poo Cleansers
Giovanni 2Chic Shampoo for Color Treated Hair
Shea Moisture Raw Shea Butter Moisture Retention Shampoo

Rinse Out Conditioner:

Aussie Moist Conditioner
Crème of Nature Argan Oil Conditioner
Herbal Essences Hello Hydration Moisturizing Conditioner
Trader Joe's Tea Tree Tingle Conditioner
Tresemme Naturals Conditioner

Deep Conditioner

Aussie Moist 3 Minute Miracle
Crème of Nature Argan Oil Intensive Conditioning Treatment
Organic Root Stimulator Olive Oil Replenishing Conditioner
Pantene Gold Series Moisture Renewal 3 Minute Miracle Deep Conditioner
Pantene Gold Series Repairing Mask
Redken Frizz Dismiss Intense Smoothing Mask
Shea Moisture Manuka Honey and Mafura Oil Intensive Hydration Masque
TGIN Honey Miracle Hair Mask

Protein Treatments

Aphogee Keratin 2 Minute Reconstructor
Brigeo Don't Despair, Repair
Olaplex Hair Perfector #3
Shea Moisture Manuka Honey and Yogurt Power Protein Treatment

Hair Oils (to be applied to wet hair)

Argan Oil
Coconut Oil-*best if used before or after shampooing*
Grapeseed Oil
Jojoba Oil
Olive Oil

Leave-In Conditioners

Cantu Shea Butter Leave-In Conditioning Cream
It's a 10 Miracle Leave-In

*Luster's S Curl No Drip Activator
Redken All Soft Mega Hydramelt Leave-In Treatment
Shea Moisture Jamaican Black Castor Oil Strengthen and Restore
Leave-In Conditioner

Anti-dandruff Shampoo

Head & Shoulders Royal Oils Co-Wash

*Product is preferred for curly or coiled hair

Extra Reading

Characteristics of Healthy Hair:
Sinclair RD. 2007. "Healthy hair: What is it?" *Journal of Investigative Dermatology*. Symposium Proceedings. Dec 1, 12(2):2–5. Elsevier.

Khumalo NP, Doe PT, Dawber RR, Ferguson DJ. 2000. "What is normal black African hair? A light and scanning electron-microscopic study." *Journal of the American Academy of Dermatology*. Nov 1, 43(5):814–20.

How Hair Products Work:
Bolduc C, Shapiro J. 2001. "Hair care products: Waving, straightening, conditioning, and coloring." *Clinics in Dermatology*. Jul 1, 19(4):431–6.

Benefits of Applying Coconut Oil to the Hair:
Gode V, Bhalla N, Shirhatti V, Mhaskar S, Kamath Y. 2012. "Quantitative measurement of the penetration of coconut oil into human hair using radiolabeled coconut oil." *Journal of Cosmetic Science*. Jan 1, 63(1):27–31.

Essential Oils for Hair Growth:
Hay IC, Jamieson M, Ormerod AD. 1998. "Randomized trial of aromatherapy: Successful treatment for alopecia areata." *Archives of Dermatology*. Nov 1, 134(11):1349–52.

The Role of Vitamin D in Hair Loss
Gerkowicz A, Chyl-Surdacka K, Krasowska D, Chodorowska G. 2017. "The role of vitamin D in non-scarring alopecia." *International Journal of Molecular Sciences*. Dec 7, 18(12):2653.

The Benefits of Caffeine on Hair Growth
Fischer TW, Hipler UC, Elsner P. 2007. "Effect of caffeine and testosterone on the proliferation of human hair follicles in vitro." *International Journal of Dermatology*. Jan, 46(1):27–35.

The Impact of Stress on Hair Loss

Hadshiew IM, Foitzik K, Arck PC, Paus R. 2004. "Burden of hair loss: Stress and the underestimated psychosocial impact of telogen effluvium and androgenetic alopecia." *Journal of Investigative Dermatology*. Sept 1, 123(3):455–7.

FDA Warning on Biotin https://www.fda.gov/medicaldevices/safety/alertsandnotices/ucm586505.htm. Accessed Apr 17, 2019.

Looking for more in depth scientific discussion of what you have read here? Then pick up my first book:

Fundamentals of Ethnic Hair: The Dermatologist's Perspective, by Drs. Crystal Aguh and Ginette Okoye

❖   ❖   ❖

Enjoyed the book? Please be sure to
visit my author page on Amazon.com to leave a positive review or
visit my website crystalaguhmd.com and leave a comment.

Made in the USA
Middletown, DE
22 September 2020